SUPERCHARGE YOUR SPERM

7 STEP PROGRAM TO BOOST YOUR FERTILITY

DR. CLARE PYERS

Cover design by: Mohammed Mudassir
Book Layout & publishing assistance by manuscript2ebook.com

Printed in Australia

TABLE OF CONTENTS

ABOUT THE AUTHOR

Clare Pyers is a Chinese Medicine Practitioner, Nutritionist, and Natural Fertility Expert who has been working in the health industry since 2001. She has worked in both mainstream and natural medicine settings, and brings a broad educational background to her practice. Her previous study includes Chemical Engineering, Chinese Medicine, Integrative Medicine and Yoga. Clare weaves all her previous knowledge, experience, and insights when working with her patients. She brings this same approach to the writing of this book.

Clare is passionate about helping people to overcome their health challenges, and believes that the best approach to holistic health incorporates strategies that identify and heal disharmonies on all levels of body, mind and spirit. She is a huge proponent of patient self-sufficiency, and loves arming her patients with the information and insights they need to be able to thrive in their health with the greatest amount of autonomy and independence possible.

When she's not writing books like this one, working with patients or running workshops - Clare loves gardening, spending time with her family and getting out into nature.

Clare lives in Melbourne, Australia with her partner and two children.

ACKNOWLEDGEMENTS

This book sat dormant in the depths of my Google drive for almost 7 years as a 95% finished draft. In this time, I lost my desire to publish it, as I endured 2 miscarriages, the birth of my second child, divorce, and 262 days of COVID lockdown in Melbourne.

It sounds like a lot, and it was at the time, but I find myself now in 2023 with a renewed sense of energy and focus. Surrounded by an almost entirely new set of friends and colleagues now, I feel incredibly supported by a fabulous bunch of people to whom I would like to give my heartfelt thanks. Without your love and reassurance and kind words, this book would have stayed hidden and might never have seen the light of day. I cannot thank you enough.

Thanks to my patients who have taught me so much over the last two decades. Thank you to my teachers and mentors whose words of wisdom continue to guide me through this wonderful journey of practising medicine. To you, the reader, for buying this book and supporting my work - I give heartfelt thanks.

Love, gratitude and thanks to Kirsten and Amy, for always assuming and knowing that writing a book is simultaneously a perfectly normal thing that people do all the time, and also a massive feat of courage, conviction and endurance.

To my darling children, Rachael and Michael, you provide me with inspiration every day as I watch you grow and develop into fine young people. Unconditional love is such a fabulous thing to give and receive. I'm so proud to be your mum. I love you both.

Most of all, thanks to Graeme, for showing me that broken hearts can mend and be loved again, for being unwavering in your strength on the days I really need you, and for supporting me 100% in all my endeavours. I love you dearly and feel so blessed to have you in my life.

INTRODUCTION

Getting pregnant is meant to be a really straightforward process. Biological imperatives. Sex makes babies. We all know that having a baby is simply a matter of making the decision and then getting down to it...right?

Many of us remember having the message of safe sex drummed into us while at high school, and possibly also from our parents. Safe sex was not just for avoiding sexually transmitted disease but also for avoiding pregnancy. Whether it was specifically said or not, most teenagers came out of those classes with the understanding that a woman can get pregnant at any time. Images were evoked of a woman's womb being like a convenience store, open for business 24 hours a day, 7 days a week, just waiting to turn your sperm into a baby.

I can certainly appreciate the value of teenagers getting a clear message about contraception, however, there is never any follow-up on this topic once we're out into our adult lives. Time passes and we are off into the workforce, we are grown up and living as adults for years, all the while holding these same beliefs that babies come too easily. We can spend years agonising over trying to avoid pregnancy at a time when we don't feel ready to become parents yet.

The tale of too-easy pregnancy can turn out to be not so straightforward as we were led to believe. It's not until we decide to start trying to conceive, and come across some problems, that we may realise the difficulties and challenges that can be part of the process.

WHO IS THIS BOOK FOR?

1 in 5 couples will have trouble conceiving. 1 in 4 pregnancies end in miscarriage. The popular line from doctors is that there's not a lot you can do for yourself to improve your odds of having a child. However, there is a lot you can do to get luck on your side, and make your baby-making project less of a gamble than a trip to the casino. You can tip the odds in your favour, by getting science on your side.

If you are thinking about trying for a baby, this book is for you. If you have already tried once or twice and you're wondering if there is something you can do to tip the odds in your favor, this book is for you. Whether you're a man or a woman, there is going to be information in this book that will be new to you, information that will be important to you on your journey towards growing your family. Yes, the title of the book and the content of the book is all about what men can do to improve their side of the equation. However, this book is designed to be read by both men and women. This book supports couples who want their relationship to not just survive, but to thrive through the process of trying to conceive. The research is inconclusive as to whether or not infertility can increase the likelihood of your marriage crumbling. However, those who have been trying for more than just a few months know just how hard the day-to-day stress that a couple experiences when they are having trouble conceiving is. It does take a toll on your relationship. I want your relationship to survive this, and to grow stronger through this process. The steps I outline in this book will help you to grow stronger as a couple as you embark on the path to reaching your fertility potential.

WORKING WITH A NATURAL MEDICINE PRACTITIONER

As a natural fertility practitioner, this book is written from my perspective, based on my clinical experience. Many people find it surprising that, despite the many benefits of following a natural medicine approach to improving your fertility, it's not well known or widely publicised that there are steps you can take before medical intervention that can help improve your fertility.

By the time someone comes to consult with a natural fertility practitioner, many people have already sought help and advice from their doctor or fertility specialist. You are often already familiar with the medical viewpoint of your fertility diagnosis, your treatment options and the chances that you will be able to fall pregnant.

The clinical opinion of a natural medicine practitioner about what is possible for you and your partner's fertility, and what can be done to improve your fertility, can be vastly different to what you have already been told.

If men are found to have sperm antibodies that are a result of a previous infection, or if there is DNA fragmentation, or poor sperm morphology, often the answer is to go to IVF because there is "nothing that can be done". Far from the truth, in fact there is a lot of published research on a range of interventions that have been shown to have a positive impact on all sperm parameters. The majority of these interventions that have been studied are nutritional medicines, including therapeutic doses of vitamins, minerals and herbal medicines. Natural medicine practitioners are the experts when it comes to determining which of these nutritional medicines are appropriate for you and designing an effective treatment regime of administering these substances. Your GP and fertility specialist are the experts at the medical aspect of treatment, and many patients successfully combine both approaches in order to increase their chances of having a baby.

When seeking the advice of a natural fertility expert, you should be looking for someone who has experience in treating fertility and who understands your full health history as well as your previous treatment history. There are many different testing procedures, drug protocols and treatment approaches that require a significant amount of knowledge of both natural and mainstream fertility treatments. Practitioners with extensive knowledge and experience in using natural medicine alongside mainstream fertility treatments can use natural medicine to further enhance your treatment outcomes. Unfortunately, without extensive knowledge and experience in the area of fertility and IVF support, a natural medicine practitioner will not necessarily have the expertise to be able to properly assess your case and determine the best treatment for you.

- They should be able to tell you about the different drug protocols and how they work in conjunction with the treatment.

- They should be able to read your blood test results, and other pathology results and provide some insight about the significance of your levels.

- They should assess your pathology results in a way that reflects optimum health by using a narrower reference range than what is provided by the laboratory.

- They should be able to tell you about their experience with the particular treatments that you have undertaken.

- They should be able to provide you with a comprehensive analysis of your health history and treatment history and ultimately, a treatment plan that can address your fertility problems.

- They should always want to assess you and your partner as a couple, because the best results come when both partners are assessed and undertake changes to optimise their fertility and enhance their overall health.

WHAT'S IN THIS BOOK?

I need to set a few things straight right from the start – this book is not about sex. I am not going to be talking about sex; there will be no critique of your sex life, fantasies or your sexuality. I'm not into telling people what they should and shouldn't be doing in the bedroom. I won't be talking about penis size, or semen retention orgasms, or tantric sex practices. Those things are not really relevant here. There's a few links at the back of the book but you can google any of this other stuff if you're interested. We're talking about what it takes to make babies, not what gets people off.

I also need to make it clear that we're not talking about your masculinity. We're not talking about how manly you feel, nor do I give any guidance or suggestions around how you need to be manlier. When we're talking about fertility, we're talking about the health of some of the smallest cells in your body – your sperm.

So, what is in this book? In my many years helping couples solve their fertility problems I've seen the same issues over and over again, and we are going to address these in this book. These issues are:

- **Men don't know that what they do with their nutrition and lifestyle to improve their overall health can also improve their fertility within a very short period of time (100 days).** In this book I will step you through the changes you can make, right down to what you eat, that will have the biggest impact. I will also discuss things you can do to help improve your overall sense of vitality, including how to improve your exercise program, deal with stress and improve your sleep habits.

- **The relationship is suffering due to the stress of trying to fall pregnant.** There are a number of ways of addressing this very common problem. You'll learn a number of approaches to changing your mindset and reinvigorating your relationship to help get out of the infertility rut.

- **The woman feels burdened with the entire responsibility for all things related to fertility and conception.** By reading this book you can help to restore some balance to this situation. You will have a game plan, with solid concrete actions you can take, that will help to better distribute the stress of trying for a baby.

- **Most men are not aware there is anything they can do to improve their sperm.** Now you know there's a whole book worth of information about things you can do that will make a real difference.

- **The information about how to improve male fertility is difficult to find.** Even within the natural fertility industry, the idea of working with male partners is still not widely discussed. Practitioners who are working to support male fertility are not well published even in the online space. Improving your swimmers takes a more coordinated and carefully structured effort than following a "Top 10 ways to improve your sperm" article written by a health blogger.

- **Male and female partners have very different thoughts and experiences around trying to conceive, and it can be a big cause of tension within the relationship.** In this book, we explore and contrast the typical mind-set and approaches taken by men and women, and offer some insights that can help to get you both singing from the same songbook.

- **There is an abundance of incorrect information that is distributed by unqualified people/poorly experienced practitioners.** I only present information that is either backed up by research or what I've found to be clinically effective with my fertility patients in-clinic. And I will also dispel some commonly held myths along the way.

- **Conventional fertility specialists have little to offer if their patients aren't responding as expected to their treatments.** Various natural medicines and an overall holistic approach are effective at improving sperm and also the chances of you taking home a baby. Whilst there is some promising research behind the majority of what I recommend to patients, almost none of it has made it into the average fertility specialist's clinical guidelines. This book is literally full of action steps that will improve your chances of responding to fertility treatment if you don't conceive naturally in the process!

This book is the result of me putting pen to paper to pull together all the knowledge and experience out of my head so I can put it into your hands. Ultimately the business of making better, faster, stronger sperm boils down to following 7 steps. These 7 steps each have a dedicated chapter where you will find all the details to help you understand what you can do and exactly why you're doing it. In brief, the 7 steps are:

Step 1: Get your head in the game

You know, part of the reason for me writing this book was prompted by seeing the massive disconnect that was happening for so many couples who were going along their fertility journey. Culturally, and historically, women do take on the majority, if not all, of the burden of fertility problems within a relationship, and they're the ones that are seeking out information, and seeking the help of doctors, specialists, and so forth.

And meanwhile, the male partner is playing a totally different game. He doesn't have a framework from which to start. There are no meaningful discussions about what's happening with sperm. There is a global decline in all sperm parameters, and it's affecting all men, some more so than others. It means that we really need to be assessing both people in the couple, and we need to be making sure that whilst we're checking out her and checking that she's okay, we need to be checking him as well. At the moment, it's a bit of an afterthought.

There's a lot of indications right from the very start of a woman's reproductive age that there could be a potential problem. Their period might be late to start. They might not get their period until they're 16, or 18 years old, or when their period does start, it could be irregular, or painful, or very heavy, or associated with problems like acne and so forth. Women often have had a lot of information about the functioning of their reproductive organs, maybe they've also had investigations and/or interventions. They have had a lot of time to come to terms with their reproductive capacity, and to question whether they want to do things to improve their reproduction. On the other hand, men don't have that same amount of feedback. They don't have anywhere near the same amount. From the age that they become sexually active, once they hit puberty, they're starting to masturbate and they're able to ejaculate. And there's an assumption that there's sperm in the ejaculate. For some men, they've never had it tested, and you wouldn't know. Men don't know that there is sperm in their ejaculate. They don't know how much is in there. They don't know how good the quality is.

The problem might not have arisen recently. It could be something that's been going on for a long time. But without the ability to measure what's going on, there is an assumption that reproductively he's fine, possibly perfect, and it coincides with all of the sexual education that happens at high school and so forth that instills the idea that a woman can get pregnant at any time.

So there is very little inclination for a man to ever consider that he may not be able to father a child. So getting your head in the game means getting onto the same page as your partner, getting onto the same program as your partner. If she's going off alcohol, if she's doing a detox, and she's exercising, she's drinking more water, you should be doing that, too. She's trying to make the best baby possible, and we want to get you into that same frame of mind. We don't want to just make a bare minimum baby. We don't want to be just doing the absolute minimum to get over the line.

It's not just about getting pregnant or not. We want you to be thinking about the quality of the sperm that you're providing to your unborn child, that's going to serve as the foundation for its health for its whole life. If you can really show her that you are on board and that you are as passionate about bringing a child into this world as she is, then that can go a really long way towards building a stronger relationship as well as optimizing your fertility and improving your health at the same time.

Step 2: What you should really be eating

Now, this is a really interesting topic because a lot of people in response to, "How's your diet?" will reply: "My diet's fine. I eat well." We're going to challenge that idea and just ask you to step it up. We don't want your diet to be fine. We want your diet to be amazing. We want your diet to have so many nutrients in it that your body is just flooded with antioxidants, minerals, and vitamins; helping to supercharge every single cell in your body. This helps not just your sperm, but also your brain, your mood, your energy levels, and every aspect of your body's functioning. We want you to be a healthy, full-of-energy man who feels as vigorous and lively as he did in his 20s, even if you're already close to or over 40 years old.

So making some key changes to your diet, which we'll outline in this stage of the program, can go a really long way to not only improving your fertility, but also optimizing your performance at work, improving your mood, improving your energy levels, and helping you to be able to live a happier life.

Step 3: Beware sperm killers

Sperm are very fragile cells. They are very sensitive to heat, they're very sensitive to pressure. You guys know how fragile your testicles and scrotum are, you don't need me or any other fertility or health expert to tell you that. You feel better if your scrotum has the space to move around unconstrained. It's not pleasant to have pressure on your groin. The reason that the scrotum is away from the body is so that it can sit at a lower temperature than the body. It's designed to sit at around 33 to 34 degrees Celsius. It's not designed to be operating at a higher temperature than that, even body temperature is too warm. And that's just the physiological aspect of easily measurable things like temperature and physical contact.

There's other things in the environment like chemicals, and toxins, that have also been proven to affect the reproductive system and in particular, to impair the ability for sperm to do their job properly. So in step six we need to be really aware of all of the factors that can impair your sperm from doing a good job. Some of these things will literally kill the sperm. Some of them will cause the sperm to be mutated. Some of them will leave the sperm slightly paralyzed and limping along. None of these things are great if you're trying to make a baby.

You need to remove as many of these things from your life as you can, and minimize your exposure to as many others as you can. We'll outline in step six exactly the actions that you need to take in order to be able to reduce your exposure to these things that are killing your sperm, and to allow your sperm to thrive and grow properly.

Step 4: Pick up heavy stuff and move it around (exercise for men)

The best thing to do for exercise in terms of building your testosterone levels is to pick up heavy things. It doesn't have to be going to the gym, but if you are going to the gym, you want to be lifting heavy weights. Building testosterone levels is directly linked with your sperm production, and the quality and quantity of sperm that you're making. So it's not to say that cardio is bad. You can still go for runs, and you can still swim, and do all of those kinds of things. But the thing that's going to make the biggest difference in your exercise program is lifting heavy weights. We'll talk about that more in step three, but we want to get that testosterone manliness energy going within your body. And that responds best to the right type of exercise.

Step 5: Stress management without the woo-woo

We've all heard that stress plays a huge role in down regulating most of the useful processes in our body, and up regulating most of the inflammatory and unhelpful processes in the body. So we know that taking care of your stress is going to be a big part of how you are able to succeed in this program.

One of the things that we do ask in terms of making changes to your diet and lifestyle, is we ask you to take out alcohol. For a lot of people, that's the only stress management tool that they have in their life. So we need to put other things into place to help you stay cool, calm, and collected, level-headed, so that you and your partner are not trying to rip each other's heads off. But we also know that you don't necessarily want to go to a meditation class and sit cross-legged chanting "Om." You don't necessarily want all the touchy-feely stuff, and I get that. So in this stage we outline some really great strategies that will make a big difference with your ability to wind down at the end of your day, and to be able to feel resilient against the stresses that come up during your daily life. And it's all stuff that leaves your masculinity intact. So head to step four to find out more about this.

Step 6: Natural medicines to supercharge your sperm

For some men, all that's required is to make some tweaks to their diet, and make some tweaks to their exercise program, and hey presto, their sperm improves. But, it all depends what your starting point is, and how much time and patience you have. We're not all created equal, and you won't all have time for a full 6 month detox to help atone for your exposures and sins. Some men have spent many years building up a tolerance to substances like alcohol, caffeine, nicotine and others. Some men have had expo-sure to certain chemicals that their body hasn't been able to detoxify properly. Some men have a genetic predisposi-tion to having more problems with their sperm than other men. Everyone has a slightly different starting point, and is working within their own parameters. Many natural medi-cines have been shown in studies to have really significant impacts on sperm quality, quantity, and motility, improving your sperm's shape and their ability to swim fast, and in the right direction.

So in this stage we go through step-by-step the details of the medicines that we commonly use in our clinic, only discussing medicines that we have found to be effective, and highlighting which medicines have also been proven in research to have good impacts on sperm.

Step 7: Staying on track

In this stage of the program we take time to reflect on how you're feeling, the improvements you've noticed, and cele-brate how well you have done to get this far.

If there are any health issues that are persisting beyond the first 30 days of the program, now is the time to take action to investigate them with your healthcare provider.

This can also be the time when complacency can start to creep in, so it's a good time to refocus your efforts and stay strong. The new habits you've created have already been imprinted into your psyche, all you need to do now is keep it up.

One of the main things that can serve as a demotivator is that, for some of you, this program is going to be really hard. I ask a lot from my patients. I ask for you to make a lot of changes. Some of these changes are huge. You may not even believe that you can make some of these changes. And it can be really difficult in that first week or two before you start really noticing the changes within yourself. It can be hard to stay motivated. I know because I walk alongside my patients every step of the way, I know it can be done, and I know you can do it.

It's really important for both of you as a couple in your fertility journey to stay on track. Making it obvious to you that what you're doing is making a difference is something that helps a lot of men in my clinic. I consider sharing these expected targets and these goals with you to be essential in helping you to stay motivated and on track, and to allow you to see for yourself and to understand the changes that are happening in your body. Remember, it's not just the sperm that we're working on. Whilst we're optimizing and improving your fertility, the nice side effect is we're also optimizing and improving every aspect of your health.

What you will find in this book is the information that my patients get when they see me in my clinic. This book is about how to get baby making working for you as a couple. It's a book about male fertility, but it's just as much a blueprint for both of you to use as you embark on this new chapter of your journey together.

Now that you've read the overview of this book and you know roughly what to expect, let's dive in and start developing your action plan to get your sperm supercharged in just 7 simple steps.

PART I:
THE FERTILITY JOURNEY

I FEEL MASCULINE. I CAN GET IT UP.
I DON'T SEE HOW THIS INVOLVES ME...

I know what you're thinking and trust me, I've heard it all before. I have seen men rolling their eyes, puffing their chests, clearing their throats and scoffing at the suggestion that they need to participate in the fertility enhancing program. Whilst there may be a global problem with sperm, it may seem like it only applies to other men but not to you. You may be feeling skeptical about the content of this book. That's ok for now. With your healthy dose of skepticism in mind, I invite you to also be curious and to approach the reading of this book with a mind that is open to possibility. Let's start at the start. Let's take a look at your overall health.

ABSENCE OF DISEASE VS HEALTH

The health of your sperm is affected by the same things that affect the health of the other cells in your body. In fact, your overall health and wellbeing is a directly measurable marker of your fertility. So, when we're talking about your fertility, we are actually talking about your overall health. So how is your health?

Maybe you think you're pretty healthy. You may think that being healthy means that you're not in hospital and you have enough energy and vitality to work a full time job without feeling like you're dying of exhaustion. Maybe you're on a medication or two, but you're feeling well since being on them so that means your health must be good. Right?

Well, it's actually not that simple. When we're talking about health, we're not talking about the absence of disease. Absence of disease and health are two very different concepts. We are talking about having all functions in your body happening in a normal and harmonious way.

Maybe you get headaches once or twice a month. They go away with a painkiller. Headaches are normal, so we would still classify you as healthy, right? Nope. Headaches are common, but they are *not* a normal part of healthy body functioning.

Maybe you eat cereal for breakfast, a sandwich for lunch, and a stir-fry for dinner. That's a pretty good diet with little room for improvement, right? Nope. Not nearly enough vegetables in that diet.

Maybe you get up at night to pee – just once though, and you get back to sleep straight away. It's because you have a glass of water with dinner a couple of hours before you go to bed. That's totally normal, and you're totally healthy, right? Nope. When your body functions optimally your lymphatic system and kidneys function at a higher level during the day and you sleep straight through until the morning without needing to pee.

There are myriad examples like this I could provide, and the purpose is not to make you feel down and miserable about your health. My goal is not to find things that are wrong with you so that I can lay blame on you for your troubles in falling pregnant. My goal is to find out where we can boost your vitality and performance across all markers of health so that we can optimize your fertility and also make you a more effective and energetic person across all aspects of your life.

Does the idea of having a close look at your health make you feel a little bit nervous?

What you will find in this book is information that will help you to not have crappy sperm. I'm known for being a straight shooter, so there won't be any sugar coating of anything in this book. If something needs to be said, I'll say it. I know you can handle that and I hope you appreciate my frank honesty. So if there is something that's not right with your health, don't sweat it, there's an action plan to follow on how to fix it, achievable to-do lists, and markers to look for on your road to awesome health.

Sperm production takes around four months from start to finish and any changes made to improve health will be directly measurable in sperm parameters. Significant improvements are possible within just a few months. Sperm quality reflects the overall state of health of a man over the previous four months.

WHY HAVEN'T I HEARD ABOUT THIS BEFORE?

How to optimize male fertility is an infrequently discussed topic. Fertility is something that a man feels is very closely linked to his sense of masculinity. Virility sits right at the core of a man's sense of manhood. This book, however, is not about how to be manlier. This book is about how to have the most awesome sperm possible. This book will show you all the necessary steps to supercharge your sperm to reach its full potential in just 7 simple steps. By following this 7-step plan to supercharge your sperm, you're doing more than just the bare minimum to get over the line when it comes to baby making.

WHY DO I NEED TO SUPERCHARGE MY SPERM?

You may currently be in one or more of the following scenarios:

- You're annoyed that sex is no longer just for fun. You're interested to find out everything you can to hurry the process along.

- You may both be feeling worn down by the unexpectedly long and difficult process of trying to conceive. You'd like to do something to help the process along and better support your partner, but you're not sure where to start or what you can do that will make a difference.

- All the logistics of trying to conceive are far too complex and complicated, and the straight-forward process of the birds and bees is not working as you expected. Honestly, at times you feel somewhat helpless, watching your partner distressed and upset. You'd like to learn more about what's going on with your fertility so that you can understand and support your partner better.

- Until reading this book you may have been feeling like a bystander in the fertility process, unaware that the changes you make will have a big impact on your fertility and chances of conceiving. Until now, nobody has told you what you can do, and you've had no plan of attack.

- You may still be in the preparation stage, and want to find out what you can do to improve your sperm before you start trying in a few months time.

No matter what stage of the fertility process you are at, there are things you can do to improve your fertility, and your overall state of health and vitality at the same time. There are things you can do that will benefit your relationship, and help to open up the communication between you. And the benefits of having a concrete plan to follow are that you can finally breathe a sigh of relief. With just a few changes, you can feel like you and your partner are working together to improve your chances of conceiving.

IT'S A GROWING PROBLEM

There is a global problem with sperm. Globally, all measurable parameters in all men have declined significantly in the past 50 years, and specifically in the past 10 to 20 years.

A semen analysis is a visual inspection by an experienced laboratory technician, and they're looking under a microscope to make a visual assessment of the sperm. The typical semen analysis looks at three main components of the sperm.

1. The count or concentration means how many actual sperm are there, and generally it's quoted in millions of sperm per milliliter.

2. The next parameter is motility. The motility describes how many of the sperm are swimming, what percentage of the sperm are swimming, and in particular, the progressive motility are the ones that are swimming in the right direction. They're not swimming around in circles, or they're not just kind of slapping their tails and not moving anywhere.

3. The third parameter is the morphology, sometimes referred to as the normal forms. This is the percentage of sperm that are the right shape, they have the right shape head, they have the right shape tails. If there is any sperm that has a defect, either in the head, or in the tail, or the mid-piece, then they are classified as being abnormally shaped.

	Laboratory Reference Ranges*	"Mr Average" 50th percentile	Top 5%
Volume	1.4ml	3ml	6.2ml
Count	15 million per ml	66 million per ml	208 million per ml
Morphology	4% normal	14% normal	39% normal
Progressive Motility	30%	55%	71%

*Lowest 5th percentile published by WHO 6th Edition

There is a startling difference in the figures in this table between the top 5% and laboratory reference ranges, and even between "Mr Average" and the laboratory reference ranges. The marker that has one of the biggest impacts is morphology. This is the measure of the shape of the sperm, and the majority of morphology problems are head defects. This means that the head of the sperm is mutated and not the right shape. Morphology is the most important factor when it comes to male fertility- the interaction between the head of the sperm and the egg is crucial to the success of the fertilisation process. If the vast majority of a man's sperm has poor morphology, it makes the chances of conception significantly lower. Poor morphology means that the majority of the sperm that make it to the egg will have physical defects that can have a negative impact on fertilisation.

4% normal morphology sperm means that 96% of them are the wrong shape. Imagine a bunch of 100 grapes that are all mouldy except for 4 or 5 grapes. When morphology is at 4%, we are seeing sperm that are produced in an environment that by and large doesn't support the production of sperm with good physical integrity. The 4% normally shaped sperm aren't necessarily great quality sperm, they're just non-deformed sperm. Taking steps to improve your health, as outlined in this book, will help to negate some of the factors that can adversely affect sperm quality and quantity and can help to improve motility.

When it comes to natural medicine, our approach is to look at all the factors that could be affecting a man's health, and therefore affecting his fertility and the sperm morphology. Unravelling any underlying health conditions helps us to improve his overall health and wellbeing and in the process improve his fertility.

A simple formula that is used in animal breeding to assess the viability of sperm is helpful to identify how much work needs to be done to get sperm powerful and dangerous.

Count x Progressive Motility % x Normal Forms % x Volume

So for our examples above with the semen reference ranges, the number of viable sperm per ejaculate:

Laboratory Reference Range = 252,000 viable sperm per ejaculate

Mr Average = 15.25 million viable sperm per ejaculate

Top 5% = 357 million viable sperm per ejaculate

When compared to 357 million per ejaculate, our baseline of 252,000 as being ok for fertility doesn't seem to reflect what men imagine in their minds when their doctor tells them their sperm is fine.

252,000 might seem like a lot of sperm, but if we look at the top 5% and see numbers that are a thousand times greater, we can see there is a lot of room for improvement even for men who are told that their sperm is fine. There's fine, and then there's awesome. This book is about helping to get you as awesome as you can be.

Of course, men don't need to have 235 million sperm in order to be able to conceive with their partner. But the higher the number of viable sperm, the higher the chances of conceiving and higher the chances that their sperm is going to have good enough stamina to not only fertilise the egg but help the embryo to be strong enough to implant and grow and become a new person.

Having the numbers can also help to measure the effects of changes that you make to your diet and lifestyle on your fertility potential. It's also useful to keep in mind that working to identify and remove the forces in your life that are impairing your fertility are the same forces that are preventing you from having over 200 million viable sperm.

PROBLEMS WITH THE WHO SEMEN GUIDELINES

One of the main problems with the WHO reference ranges is that the information is not necessarily useful in helping you to get a clear perspective on your fertility. The World Health Organization releases guidelines that are used by laboratories and reproductive specialists around the world to be able to assess the likelihood of sperm being able to fertilize an egg and support life.

A big part of the problem is that nowadays these parameters are not necessarily in line with what is required for natural conception to occur, and men can get a false impression of their fertility. The lower limit of the current parameters can give an indication of the likelihood of a good outcome from assisted reproductive technology such as IVF. Having two or three of these parameters slightly above the reference range can result in a man being told that he is fertile when, in actual fact, he does have impaired fertility. Without having 2 or more sperm parameters well above the current reference ranges it's very unlikely that natural conception will occur.

The parameters mean that sperm can be classified as "normal" or "fine" despite 95% of your sperm being the wrong shape, with less than half of them swimming in the right direction, and only 15 million sperm per ml (when ideally we would normally like to see well over 100 million per ml). If your sperm falls within these guidelines, your sperm can be classified as fine, when 20 years ago it would have qualified for a diagnosis of triple factor male infertility.

There are three main problems the current WHO guidelines for semen analysis:

1. Reference ranges are changing to reflect the average man.

2. Reference ranges are now more reflective of what will support fertility in conjunction with the highest intervention assisted reproductive technology.

3. There is a global free-fall in sperm parameters and there is evidence that poor sperm quality is not only linked with a range of fertility problems but also increases a man's risk of other problems such as testicular cancer. Despite this, few men are told that their sperm might be the problem, and even fewer men are given information or support about what they can do to improve it.

In my clinic we have seen many cases of infertility where a couple has been given all kinds of female reproductive diagnoses as their reason for not conceiving – *despite the sperm parameters being clearly outside the reference range* – including:

- unexplained infertility
- endometriosis
- Polycystic Ovarian Syndrome (PCOS)
- "old eggs" or ovarian failure

Women are often left to unnecessarily shoulder the burden of the blame and guilt that comes along with not being able to conceive. Often the woman puts in considerable effort to try to correct things like endometriosis or PCOS, only to find once their problems are resolved that there has been a problem with the sperm all along. I have worked with many couples who have been diagnosed as having egg quality issues, who have spent tens or even hundreds of thousands on treatment using donor eggs only to find that their "old" poor quality eggs fertilised just fine with donor sperm.

Spending time to get the right diagnosis at the start, can result in quicker action to focus your efforts, attention and resources to addressing the true problem.

GETTING THROUGH IT TOGETHER

One of the most common problems a couple experiences if they are having trouble conceiving is the strain it puts on their relationship. There is a lot of pressure to get the timing right; to be having sex when you don't necessarily feel in the mood for it; the two week wait where the woman feels like every sensation in her body is a potential sign of pregnancy.

MYTH ABOUT MALE SEXUALITY : ALWAYS UP FOR IT

Male potency and virility are associated in our culture with a man's ability to obtain and sustain an erection, and to be able to sexually "satisfy" and impregnate his partner. The stereotype that all men are ready, willing, and able to engage in sexual activity at any time or any place have contributed to unrealistic expectations regarding sexual functioning in men.

FERTILITY PROBLEMS AND RELATIONSHIP BREAKDOWN

Statistically, if you don't end up having a child together your relationship is more likely to end. For some couples the heartache of not being able to conceive creates an irreparable divide between them that results in the complete breakdown of their relationship. This is even more likely to occur if IVF doesn't work.

Ultimately, one of the biggest problems that occurs during a couple's fertility journey is that they become disconnected from one another.

Mentally and emotionally, the process of trying to make a baby feels different for a man than it does for a woman.

Physically, the process of trying to make a baby is very different for a man and a woman.

From a cultural point of view, it's automatically considered to be a female issue if a couple is having difficulty conceiving. This harks back to the time of Henry VIII who had many wives, the majority of whom were beheaded for being "barren". If they were able to conceive they had repeated miscarriages; some children were born but were so unwell they didn't live more than a week or two. Rather than seeing that he was the common denominator in the equation where eight women were unable to conceive using his seed, each of these women were declared as barren, a crime they paid for with their lives. This part of history is known to many, but the part that isn't well reported is that Henry VIII suffered with extremely poor health and this was the contributing factor to the infertility he experienced with each of his wives. While not confirmed, he has been suspected of having syphilis, uncontrolled diabetes, and growth hormone deficiency; he also had pus filled boils on his skin and was suspected of suffering from gout. Despite these factors, culturally it was still considered to be the woman's burden to bear if she couldn't become pregnant and give birth to a healthy child.

The modern day version of this sentiment is peddled with the idea that women have "old eggs" and that beyond a certain age it is all reliant on the woman as to whether or not a couple will conceive. "Nothing to be done" is the main idea that resides in our culture when it comes to men, and the idea that masculinity, virility and fertility are intertwined makes it difficult for these conversations to start. There is evidence for paternal age playing a role in a range of fertility problems; together with the recent decline in sperm parameters there is even more reason why we should be talking more about what a couple can do about their fertility, rather than what a woman can do.

PROBLEMS IN THE BEDROOM

Rather than being spontaneous, initiated by desire, and focused on enjoying the intimacy, what often happens when a couple is trying to conceive is that their sex life becomes a precise, clinical series of encounters that often lack spontaneity, desire, intimacy and overall enjoyment.

Resentment sets in.

Getting "the nudge" no longer excites you, in fact for some men it can make them feel like they are being used as a sperm donor.

Certain positions are considered to be more successful than others in conceiving. According to Google, there are many before, during and after sex rituals that need to be performed. From your woman propping herself up after sex and doing bicycle legs in the air, to the pressure of timing orgasms for just the right moment so that her cervix can dip down and scoop up your semen at the very moment you ejaculate. Having special lube, or no lube. Or using egg whites as lube (as one naturopath suggested on their blog) and praying it doesn't turn to scrambled eggs.

Sex on demand can cause all kinds of problems both within the relationship but also for performance. It's not uncommon for so many emotional upsets to be going on within the relationship and within the bedroom dynamic that the pressure leaves men struggling to get and maintain an erection, and then struggle further to even be able to ejaculate.

And we thought it was a problem that no one was talking about male infertility? When it comes to infertility based performance problems, it's a huge problem and we're *really* not talking about that, are we?

Couples will often deal with the stress of fertility problems in different ways. The disconnect that lies underneath many of the stresses of fertility issues can arise from the different philosophical approaches each person has about the challenges in their unique situation. Whether it's the financial strain of IVF, pressure and inappropriate comments and questions from friends and family, the grief of losing a pregnancy - if you aren't both on the same page about the significance of the issue and the best way to move through the stress, it can create distance between the two of you.

And that translates to distance in your sex life.

Instead of sex being about connecting with each other, sharing intimacy, it can become a reminder of the failure of your repeated attempts to conceive.

"As human beings, we are sexual beings and it is imperative that we don't trade our sexuality for our fertility"

Beth Jaeger-Skigen, Couples therapist

Advice on what to do to help strengthen your sex life during this difficult time:

- Starting working on your sex life now. Don't put it on the To-Do list for after you're pregnant, or after you've finished your family. Your sex life may be different during the time that you're trying to conceive but it doesn't have to be unsatisfying or non-existent.

- Consider having sex outside of your fertile times as a way to help reconnect and remind yourselves of the pleasure, connection and intimacy you can give and receive from each other.

- Know that you're not alone. It is really common for couples to experience significant disruption to their sex life during prolonged periods of trying to conceive. Dramatic changes to your sex life is a very common response to the stress you as a couple are facing during this time.

- Focus on ways to reconnect and be intimate with each other that don't involve having sex. Go to a couples workshop or couples retreat, or take a weekend getaway to a romantic destination. Focus on rediscovering each other's bodies, cuddle, massage, erotic touch. Take sex off the table and focus on making each other feel good.

- Consider seeing a therapist if you feel like you need to have additional help and support to reconnect with each other.

YOU'RE IN THIS TOGETHER

Regardless of who needs to work more on their health and fertility, and who may or may not be dragging the other partner across the line – you are in this journey together. You and your partner, either alone or together, will attend many appointments throughout your fertility journey with your GP, fertility specialist or natural medicine practitioner, you will undergo a barrage of testing and subject yourselves to the ongoing cycles of fertility supportive interventions.

You may or may not end up with a baby out of all this. No fertility program on the planet can prove a 100% success rate. However, at the end of all this there will be the two of you, and the strength of your relationship will be one of the factors that will determine if you have the stamina to endure the changes you'll need to implement and the effort you will both need to put towards this project of making another human being. I've seen many couples over the years go through the process of trying to conceive, and I've seen the greatest success with couples who are both fully on board. This means that I've worked with both the man and the woman for several months to get their health and fertility optimised. They've both fully taken on board the nutrition changes, the lifestyle changes, are both taking their herbal medicine and having acupuncture, they're exercising, and they're focusing on communicating well, connecting with each other and re-establishing or building on their intimacy, both in sexual and non sexual ways.

On the other end of the spectrum, sometimes I'm working with a woman and I hear about her husband. I might see his semen analysis results if he's had one done, but I might never meet him. She comes to my office in tears of distress that he's out drinking, or out partying and taking drugs with his mates. Or that she can't get him to have sex with her during her fertile times. There are many distraught and unhappy women out there who are living in a very different universe than the one their partner lives in. They can't connect properly with each other; she's pissed off, frustrated and resentful about his lack of interest or dedication in attempting to conceive. He's pissed off, frustrated and resentful that there's so much pressure and expectation being put onto him. Sometimes he doesn't really want a baby. Sometimes he's just scared about the realities of being able to provide for a family, and is scared about growing up and taking that next life step. I don't ever really get to find out what is exactly going on in the minds of these men because I don't get to meet them.

Many times, the dynamic of a couple's relationship lies somewhere between the two extremes. The male partner has some level of interest in supporting his partner on their fertility journey but doesn't really own his possible role in the process. There's no established dialogue within our culture to support men undergoing fertility support, and there's barely a dialogue around supporting women undergoing fertility treatment because it's still something that's shrouded in secrecy, shame and private suffering. We sometimes think that if an intervention is powerful enough to change the course of our destiny and potential outcome, it would be reported on the news or someone would tell us about it..

I'm that someone that is opening up the dialogue. This is why I'm writing this book, to provide support to the people who need it the most. For the couples who are struggling with what to do next to improve their chances of falling pregnant. For the women who desperately need to show their man that he can actually be the hero in all of this, in a way that supports his feelings of masculinity, and help him feel stronger and more connected with his partner along the way. For the men who are sitting on the sidelines watching the stress of the fertility process take a toll on their partner but have been provided with no other medical support or advice, other than statistics, the advice to try every month, and possibly needing to hand over their credit card for a clinical medical approach with a 28% success rate if the wait-and-see approach doesn't work.

This book is primarily written as a resource for the men out there, a manual to help guide you through the ins-and-outs of boosting your fertility and strengthening all aspects of your health and relationship along the way. But it's also a valuable guide for women as well, to help them understand the process and the issues their partner may be experiencing.

You're in this together, and so a large part of the reason why I've written this book is to provide a couple with the framework to be able to take this journey together. So that your relationship doesn't end up as just another statistic of infertility and disintegrate or suffer as a result.

What I want for you as a couple is to embark on this journey together and to use it as a way to strengthen your relationship and deepen the bonds between you so that you can walk along the path together and not feel alone. I want you to be able to align yourselves on all levels, not just with the desire to start trying to conceive a baby, and not just with the ideas that you might have around how you're going to raise the child. Can you imagine how good it would feel for you both to get totally onto the same page? All the logistics and all the finer details of what's going to be involved to get your bodies ready, who better to take the journey with than the person who will be co-parenting with you in the years to come?

Take this journey together. Through the preparation period. Through the preseason of being able to get your bodies in tiptop shape. Get your minds and your hearts aligned on this project together.

One of the benefits of doing this is that your relationship becomes stronger and more able to withstand the challenge of adversity. So that if it does eventuate that you're not able to conceive a child, or you're not able to get pregnant, and you're not able to expand your family in the way that you would have hoped, your relationship is far more likely to be able to withstand this challenge.

I can't guarantee that you're going to come out the other side of this process with a baby in your hands. Nobody can provide you with that guarantee. What I can assure you is that, if the two of you embark on this project together and you wholeheartedly take on board all of the things that I've outlined in this book, that not only will you feel fitter, stronger, happier and healthier, but your relationship will also be stronger as well.

EVERYONE ELSE IS PREGNANT, WHY AREN'T WE?

To help you fully understand and navigate this difficult problem, it's important for you to first have realistic expectations about how long it might take you and your partner to conceive, and the factors that influence this timeframe.

HOW LONG SHOULD IT TAKE TO GET PREGNANT?

If a couple has no fertility problems, they will conceive within 3 months on average. There is no need to wait for 12 months before a visit to investigate possible medical issues is needed. Mainstream medical consensus says that couples under the age of 35 should be investigated after 12 months of not conceiving whilst having unprotected intercourse, and 6 months for couples over the age of 35. Generally this involves a visit to a fertility specialist, and investigations and treatments that determine the type of fertility treatment you're likely to need. However, it doesn't mean you need to go to IVF straight away either. There is a missing step in between starting to try to conceive, and going to IVF when that doesn't work. The in-between step is to take action to improve your reproductive health, and that can be done in as little as 8-12 weeks.

HOW YOUR HEALTH AFFECTS CONCEPTION TIMEFRAMES

If both the man and woman have full 5 star health, there will usually be no delay in being able to conceive.

What does five star health look like?

When people talk about the idea of being healthy, they often imagine themselves as being free of disease. Whilst being free of disease is a good pre-requisite for optimum health or five star health, being in optimum health involves far more than just lacking a disease or lacking an illness.

Optimum health looks a little bit like this: **your energy levels are high**. You wake up in the morning and you feel vibrant and ready to start the day. Your energy doesn't fade, or wax and wane after meals or due to stress and you have enough energy to be able to do all of the things that you'd like to do in your day.

You, of course, feel tired by the end of the day, but you're not falling asleep on the couch at 7:00pm at night. You have enough energy to be able to eat your dinner and socialize with your family before going to bed.

RED FLAG: You don't have enough energy to get through your day

OPTIMAL: Your sleep, when you're in optimum health, is restful. You fall asleep easily and you're able to stay asleep. You don't wake up in the middle of the night to visit the bathroom or to roll over. You're not easily woken by noises or the other person who you're sharing a bed with every time they roll over or cough. You're not disturbed by your dreams. Whilst you might dream and you might remember your dreams in the morning, they don't affect your quality of sleep and you wake in the morning feeling rested.

RED FLAG: You aren't able to get 7-8 hours of unbroken sleep.

OPTIMAL: Your digestion has no problems at all. You wake up in the morning hungry and ready for breakfast. You don't have any particular problems with digesting any particular sorts of foods. You don't get bloated after eating. You don't have reflux. You are able to tolerate a wide variety of foods without it affecting your skin or your mood or your energy levels. Your bowels are functioning well and you have a bowel movement at least once a day. It's formed and it's not loose or too hard or difficult to pass. You don't have any problems with hemorrhoids or bleeding from the bowel.

RED FLAG: You have reflux, loose bowels, rectal bleeding or cramping.

OPTIMAL: Your skin is in good health. It's not dry, it's not too oily. You don't have any rashes or any problems like eczema or dermatitis or psoriasis.

RED FLAG: You have problem skin. You have used roac-cutane (acne medication) in the past.

OPTIMAL: You don't suffer from headaches and you don't remember the last time that you needed to take a pain-killer for a headache. Your thirst is healthy and you can easily drink two liters of water per day without feeling water-logged or without forgetting to drink water.

RED FLAG: You have one or more spontaneous headaches each month.

OPTIMAL: Your appetite is strong and healthy. You don't have aversions or cravings for any particular types of food, and you don't have anything that happens within your body on a regular basis that can impair or reduce your appetite for eating.

RED FLAG: You skip meals, or forget to eat because of low appetite.

OPTIMAL: Your body is free from aches and pains. You don't have any aching in your lower back or knees or ankles, and you don't suffer from any types of arthritis or stiffness in your joints at all.

RED FLAG: You have aching in your lower back or knees.

OPTIMAL: Your mood is healthy and whilst you might regularly experience a free flowing range of all the emotions, you don't get stuck in one particular type of emotion such as anger or frustration or resentment. You're able to experience and express happiness, sadness, anger, grief, worry and contentment without any problems.

RED FLAG: You are taking antidepressant or antianxiety medication. You have strong negative emotions that regularly dominate the way you feel.

Of course, we're talking about fertility, and so we need to talk about your reproductive health as well. For men and women, a healthy libido is an indication of good health, although it's not uncommon for couples to experience changes in their libido if they have been trying to conceive for a while.

For women, we also look at the menstrual cycle and a healthy woman in optimum health is going to have a period that comes regularly every 28 to 29 days. She's going to bleed for five to six days. There will be **no pain** at all. There will be no discomfort, **no symptoms leading up to the period** of breast tenderness, moodiness, fatigue, appetite changes, fluid retention and the other myriad symptoms that are often classified as being PMS or premenstrual syndrome. **There is literally no fanfare around her monthly period, other than that she bleeds for five days**.

Of course, for fertility it's required for a woman as well to have a good level of estrogen and also of follicle stimulating hormone and luteinizing hormone that help to ripen and release an egg. This is demonstrated in a woman by a discharge from her vagina at around the middle of her cycle, that coincides with ovulation. In a woman who is in optimal health, this period of fertile discharge will last around three to five days. The levels of these markers can be confirmed with a blood test from your GP or your fertility specialist.

In men, reproductive health is demonstrated by the ability to **achieve and sustain an erection**. Even in men who have performance issues, there's always going to be, in a healthy man, a physiological ability to have an **erection first thing in the morning** when they wake up, unrelated to sexual desire or arousal.

If one partner has no fertility red flags and the other has one or two fertility red flags, there may be a delay in being able to conceive but could potentially be able to conceive on their own. It will most likely take longer than normal, up to 12–18 months.

If both partners have one or two fertility red flags, there is a chance they won't be able to conceive unless they seek help to improve their fertility. Many cases of unexplained infertility fall into this category, where both partners have small problems with their fertility but combined it can be a barrier to conceiving.

If one partner has three or more fertility red flags, they probably won't be able to conceive naturally and may also not have success with assisted reproduction techniques such as IVF and ICSI. They generally need to make improve-ments to their health to lift their fertility into a state where they will be able to conceive either naturally or with IVF.

If both partners have three or more fertility red flags, there is a chance they won't be able to conceive even with assistance.

COMMON CAUSES OF FERTILITY PROBLEMS

Fertility problems are becoming more and more common, with many couples now having difficulty conceiving in a normal timeframe of 12 months. Many factors are at play, the main ones being:

- Couples are waiting until later in life to start a family.

- The health of the general population is declining. This plays a big role in fertility.

- Common nutritional deficiencies that result from a poor diet or a malabsorption syndrome can result in poor sperm production, imbalanced hormones, interrupted or absent ovulation, and irregular menstruation.

- Endocrine disrupting chemicals are everywhere in our homes and workplaces and magnify hormonal imbalances.

- Emotional health and wellbeing is in decline, as stress and mental health problems continue to increase each year. This affects the proper functioning of the hormonal reproductive system.

- Even if they are fertile, women are sometimes unsure if they are ovulating each month, or exactly when their fertile period might be occurring.

- All measurable parameters of sperm quality have declined dramatically in the past 15 years, with falling quality and quantity continuing to occur in men throughout the world.

- The stress, anxiety and pressure around trying to conceive puts a lot of pressure on relationships and can bring resentment and reluctance into a couple's sex life.

- There are an increasing number of couples each year who are diagnosed with unexplained infertility.

By correcting any of these barriers, and visiting a natural medicine practitioner who specialises in treating fertility, most couples can conceive naturally. Additionally, after addressing all the above barriers, and working with a practitioner to achieve optimum health, couples who are unable to conceive naturally are more likely to conceive with the help of IVF or ICSI.

YOU MAY HAVE BEEN TOLD YOU NEED IVF WHEN YOU ACTUALLY DON'T

We see a lot of people in our clinic who are seeking assistance to improve their fertility to conceive naturally, or to improve their chances of IVF and ICSI resulting in pregnancy. *What they are actually seeking is help to expand their family with the birth of a healthy child.*

What some people don't realise is that fertility problems can be an opportunity in disguise. By working to improve their overall health, it's more likely their epigenetics will be improved. This means that good genes are more likely to be switched on and bad genes are more likely to be switched off. The woman who has balanced her hormones and improved her digestion will have a happier environment in her body for her baby to develop in, giving the baby the optimal conditions for good health. There is a lot of research linking pre-conception and peri-natal (the period immediately before and after birth) nutrition to all kinds of health outcomes, and showing that making changes during the pre-conception and peri-natal period can have a positive impact on the child's health. Sadly, there is also research linking IVF and assisted reproduction with poor health outcomes for the child. It's my belief that this is not necessarily as a direct result of the IVF procedure itself, and that the same epigenetic improvements you can get from improving your overall health and your sperm can also help to avoid some of these poor health outcomes being passed onto your child.

Improving health before conceiving is important for supporting the wellbeing of your child, and for many couples will result in conception happening naturally. However, there are some commonly held beliefs and faulty thinking that lead people to think that not much can be done about their fertility, and if they can't conceive naturally then going to IVF will solve all problems. There is also a belief that doctors know everything there is to know about natural fertility treatments and supportive measures you can take to improve your fertility, and that your doctor will recommend all options that could benefit you.

GPs are generalist doctors, and they know a lot about a lot of topics, everything needed to tend to your basic needs, and the knowledge of knowing when to refer to a specialist. They don't have training in natural medicine, and it's not part of their clinical practice guidelines in Australia to be routinely referring to a natural medicine practitioner. Recent changes in code of practice for GPs in Australia have made the guidelines around a GP referring to a non-mainstream health provider very strict. A referral to a natural fertility specialist is not as likely as you might expect.

Fertility specialists are highly specialised doctors, and their training is in scientific, medical treatments including testing and diagnosis, surgery and medications. Very few fertility specialists have undertaken further study in the use of herbal medicines and supplements for supporting fertility. Unfortunately they are therefore not in a position to be able to prescribe these to you, or to necessarily even know what the potential benefits are.

Many patients share with me that they are disappointed their GP or their fertility specialist didn't recommend they incorporate natural medicine into their fertility treatment sooner. Especially when there is a growing body of evidence for many of the routinely prescribed supplements and herbal medicines for supporting all parameters of male and female fertility. Many patients also share with me their disappointment at the lack of support their GP or fertility specialist shows towards their natural medicine treatment, or even their dismay when they are instructed by their specialist to stop taking their prescribed herbal medicines or supplements due to the specialist not having enough information about how they work.

As a natural medicine practitioner who has a fertility focused practice, prescribing herbal medicines and supplements to support your fertility is something I do every day in the clinic. It's part of my job to understand how they work, to understand the way that they may or may not interact with your existing medications, to be aware of the risks, the potential side effects and how to monitor for clinical effectiveness. Often there are things we can do with natural medicine that are not widely known or accepted as being possible by mainstream medicine. This is especially true when it comes to supporting male fertility. We can help to improve many of your sperm parameters with a comprehensive program of diet, exercise, herbal medicines and supplements.

If it's the case that we can improve your sperm, it's also the case that we can improve your fertility and increase your chances of being able to conceive naturally. Improvements that occur in your sperm parameters could mean the difference between you and your partner being able to conceive naturally vs believing that your only option is IVF. If your partner doesn't have any significant reproductive issues like blocked fallopian tubes or endometriosis, following this program and improving your sperm could save you thousands by help you conceive naturally, or reduce the number of IVF cycles you will need to be able to conceive and welcome your baby into the world.

RISK OF MISCARRIAGE

If you have suffered pregnancy loss in the past, you know that it can be a very traumatic and upsetting experience. Often the pregnancy has been lost before a woman has shared her news with family and friends, and many women grieve alone during this time. The medical viewpoint that normalises miscarriage and tells couples that miscarriage is so common as to almost be expected, doesn't necessarily offer a couple much comfort during this time.

There are a range of preventable factors that can contribute to miscarriage risk. Similarly, there are a range of factors that can support a pregnancy to become fully established, with the embryo being able to grow fully and be born as a baby nine months later. From a male fertility point of view, it's not simply a matter of your sperm being able to fertilise the egg and "job done". There are sperm factors that can play a role in miscarriage including:

- Chromosomal problems and DNA integrity of the sperm
- Mitochondrial energy production

Up to 50% of miscarriages are related to genetic and chromosomal problems. This is often due to additional chromosomes either in the egg or the sperm. It's important to do as many things as possible to reduce the risk of DNA fragmentation in your sperm, and to maintain the integrity of your sperm and its mitochondrial energy production. Outlined in this program are actions you can take to improve the quality of your sperm and reduce the risk of miscarriage.

WHEN AND HOW OFTEN SHOULD WE HAVE SEX?

U nlike the spiel we give to teenagers, it's not true that having sex at any time in a woman's cycle will lead to pregnancy. There are many biological processes that need to occur in unison in order for pregnancy to begin, thankfully most of those processes occur without us needing to worry about them. The real window in a woman's cycle for being able to conceive is only around 3-5 days, and there are some tricks to being able to reliably monitor when that fertile window is active.

THE FERTILE WINDOW

Luteinising hormone (LH) is one of the hormones that stimulates ovulation. In the presence of high estrogen levels, LH and follicle stimulating hormone (FSH) will prompt the ovaries to release a mature egg. LH also stimulates the mucous cells of the cervix; normally throughout the month a mucous "plug" is in place that provides a barrier between the uterus and the outside world. During the time when LH is active, the mucous cells are stimulated and the mucous plug will shift as the cervix opens. Generally a 3-5 day timeframe leading up to ovulation is when you will be able to notice changes in vaginal discharge. The nature of the cervical mucus changes to become more slippery, and this tells you when a woman is approaching ovulation. When the mucus plug is released, the cervix is open, and this means her baby-making factory is open for business. Once the fertile discharge is observed, this is the fertile window and the time when conception can occur.

Generally a woman will also experience a peak in her libido at this time of the month. If there are fewer than three days of obvious wet fertile mucus at this time of the month it can reflect an underlying hormonal imbalance in the woman that in many cases is enough to prevent pregnancy from occurring. An experienced natural fertility expert will be able to identify what is happening and put a program in place to improve her fertility.

Fertile window when conception can occur:

- Slippery profuse vaginal discharge
- Increase in her libido
- Occurs over a 3-5 day window prior to ovulation

Have sex as often as you like in this time if you want to conceive.

Once the egg is released, it only survives 12-24 hours if not fertilised in time. It's important for the sperm to be there ready and waiting for the egg before the egg is released, or get there as soon as possible after the egg is released in order for there to be enough time for fertilisation to occur. It's a long swim from the cervix to the end of the fallopian tube, so ideally you have been having regular sex every day or every second day leading up to ovulation. This allows the sperm enough time to get into position, so they are ready and waiting at the ovary to fertilise the egg when it's released. The fertile mucus present in the vagina and the cervix serves to preserve the sperm, and acts like a superhighway for the sperm, helping to support their successful journey to the ovaries. Anytime there is fertile mucus present in the vagina, this is a sign that the mucus plug is gone, and that the womb is "open for business". Whether this occurs on day 9, or day 19 of a woman's menstrual cycle, there is an opportunity for the sperm to penetrate into the womb and the fallopian tubes in preparation for the release of the egg.

Once the egg is fertilised it's referred to as an embryo, and it then takes around 7-10 days for it to travel to the uterus and implant into the lining of the womb.

HOW OFTEN SHOULD WE BE HAVING SEX?

Ideally, a couple's sex life is based on desire and attraction. Unfortunately, one of the biggest complaints reported by couples having trouble conceiving is that there is so much pressure tied to the logistics of getting it right that the enjoyment and pleasure of sex is very quickly destroyed. She is madly peeing on ovulation test sticks, or spitting onto a microscope slide and trying to work out if she's fertile. You are standing by, not really too sure if you can do anything to help, until her fertile window rolls around where you often are left simply feeling like a sperm donor who is expected to perform on demand.

As soon as a woman notices the start of her fertile mucus, this indicates that her fertile window has begun. This is the best time to have intercourse, and you can have sex as often or as infrequently during this period as you like. Provided the woman's fertile window has been accurately identified, once is enough, multiple times is totally fine if that is your preference. Once ovulation has been confirmed (by basal body temperature charting indicating her post ovulation hormonal shift has happened) then the fertile window is closed again. From now until the end of her cycle, you can both just continue to have sex as your desire dictates.

A common question I am asked is: is it possible to have sex too often? This is often prompted by conflicting advice of having sex every second day throughout the women's cycle, versus the advice of having sex every day during the fertile window, and people feeling like it can be easy to get it wrong. My advice to my patients is that as long as they have sex at least once during the fertile window, they are doing the minimum required to achieve pregnancy. If having sex more often is detrimental emotionally to your connection with each other, or leaves one of you feeling tired and depleted, I don't recommend having sex just for the sake of it. Men especially can feel quite depleted if they are having sex every day, whilst also having to work long hours, alongside other commitments like exercise or hobbies. Women tend not to experience such a lull in energy around ovulation, and tend to experience the largest upswing in their libido and feel more energised at this time of their cycle.

It is possible to have sex too infrequently, this is especially the case for a man who has poor sperm morphology. If the normal sperm count is below 10%, I advise my patients to keep their sperm regularly turning over, to encourage the production of new sperm and reduce debris and white blood cells and other accumulations that can reduce a man's fertility. Ideally a man with low sperm morphology will be ejaculating at least every second day from the start of a woman's menstrual cycle to help promote better morphology leading up to the woman's fertile window. During non fertile times it is totally up to the preference of the couple, and it doesn't matter if this is achieved either through intercourse or masturbation. During the woman's fertile window the ejaculation should continue every second day - ideally this means the couple is having sex every second day throughout this time.

WHAT'S GOING ON WITH SPERM?

With almost every couple I've worked with, where there was a problem with the sperm, they were initially told that the sperm was fine. This is occurring even more frequently due to changes in the reference ranges from most laboratories, as discussed below.

One of the biggest things to change over the past 10-15 years is the quality of sperm produced by the average male. Many theories exist about the cause(s) of this phenomenon, but one thing for sure is that all markers of sperm quality have declined dramatically in a very short period of time.

MEASURING SPERM QUALITY

The table in chapter 3 shows the sperm parameters given by the World Health Organisation as a benchmark to be used by laboratories to assess sperm quality, and shows how these parameters have changed over the past 15+ years. These represent the standard or "average" man, and it's easy to see that the standard of normal sperm has deteriorated quite dramatically over the past 20-30 years. The past 20-30 years has also seen worldwide increased utilisation of assisted reproductive technologies in conjunction with this decline in male fertility.

SPERM QUALITY AND BEING OVERWEIGHT

The link between obesity and infertility is especially relevant for men with a BMI above 32 kg/m^2. Men who are overweight or obese are more likely to have less sperm overall, less of that sperm is likely to be swimming in the right direction, more of those sperm will have abnormal shape, and the DNA within the sperm itself is more likely to be damaged.

- Lower sperm count
- Lower sperm motility
- Lower normal morphology (shape)
- Increased DNA fragmentation

Testicular oxidative stress is known to play a big role, essentially this is what happens when your body can't get rid of the by-products of normal physiological functioning. Instead of your body being able to get rid of the waste products, they accumulate and cause damage to the sperm cells and DNA within the sperm.

Men who are overweight or obese are also more likely to have higher levels of estrogen, and lower levels of testosterone. This has direct effects on the body's ability to produce good quality sperm, as well as system-wide effects that increase risk of a range of diseases including cancer and heart disease.

SPERM QUALITY AND CANCER

What hasn't been hinted at in these test results is that sperm quality is a reflection of the health of the man, and infertility is linked with increased rates of reproductive cancers in men. I recommend to any man without hesitation that if he has any sperm parameters outside the normal range, that it might be a good idea to do something about his fertility– regardless of whether the couple wants to conceive naturally or use medical assistance. Taking action to normalise semen parameters will help to reduce his risk of reproductive cancer and other serious diseases.

Poor fertility and semen and sperm abnormalities are associated with an increased risk of testicular and prostate cancer. Even if you decide that you don't want to pursue changes to improve your fertility, your risk for cancer still remains. Having abnormal sperm increases your risk of cancer. Sperm is a marker for your overall health and well-being, and is a product of the state of your health over the preceding 100 days or so. Making changes to your health and to optimise your fertility not only increases your chances of being able to conceive, it also increases the chances you're going to be around to see those children grow up and have children of their own.

And if making changes helps you to be able to conceive without the need for IVF then you are also reducing your partner's risk of ovarian cancer – which is increased if she undergoes IVF. Women undergoing IVF treatment have a 30% increased chance of developing ovarian cancer than women who haven't done IVF treatment. Ovarian cancer is still a cancer that is associated with a high mortality rate, as it often has very vague symptoms or no symptoms at all until it's in the later stages.

I recommend making as many changes as possible to improve your health so that you're more likely to conceive naturally, or if you go to IVF you're more likely to conceive with fewer attempts – leaving you both with a reduced risk of these reproductive cancers than you would otherwise have.

SIMPLE CHANGES CAN HAVE A BIG IMPACT

The good news in all this is that sperm only takes around 3 months to be made from start to finish, and overall, reflects the man's general state of health during that time. Any changes that are made to improve overall health and well-being will contribute to improving all sperm parameters and include:

- going on a detox
- drinking more water
- cutting out coffee and alcohol
- eating more vegetables
- reducing body fat and losing weight

Sperm are highly susceptible to environmental factors like stress, endocrine disrupting chemicals, poor nutrition and overwork. What has happened to sperm in the past 15 years is a reflection in the decline of health of the average man. We see this reflected in the drastic drop in laboratory semen parameters, to the point where now a man can be classified as having no fertility issues when he has very few sperm, more than half of his sperm aren't swimming and 97% of his sperm are misshapen and disfigured.

Because sperm is produced quite quickly, it is relatively receptive to changes in diet, lifestyle and nutrition. Making some simple changes can have a big impact on the quality of sperm, and subsequently on the chances of a couple conceiving, and having a healthy child. Throughout the rest of this book we will outline in detail the changes you can implement to give you the best chances of improving your sperm.

PROTECTING YOUR LIFE ESSENCE

The Chinese medicine philosophy talks about the sperm as reflecting the quality of life essence of the man; a woman's eggs reflect the quality of her life essence. We inherit our life essence from our parents. It is a potent life force that is gradually used up as we live our lives, and when it runs out, we die. Through proper diet and lifestyle we can protect the life essence from being overused. Rather than running on empty and using up our reserves, we can be nourished with good food and nutrition and get adequate rest to restore vitality. Living a stressful life and having inadequate nutrition and rest forces your body to chew through its reserves in order to continue functioning. The old saying "Live fast, die young" can be one way of interpreting what happens when you spend your life essence too quickly.

So how can you go about protecting your life essence? Do the opposite of live fast, die young!

- going to bed early, waking up with the sun

- eat moderately - adequate but not excessive amounts

- move your body - adequately but not excessively

- regulate your emotional landscape, don't get stuck in mental loops, let your stress go at the end of your day

- do things each day that you enjoy

Essentially what this translates to is a checklist of "living in accordance with nature" factors, consisting of diet and lifestyle advice that promote good physical and mental health, emotional resilience and hormonal balance.

HAVING YOUR SPERM TESTED

C hances are if you're reading this book, you're already well down the road to trying for a baby. At the very least, you're actively planning to start trying soon.

Did you know it's a standard thing for a woman to go and get some routine blood tests done before trying to get pregnant to make sure certain things are in order?

If you're a numbers man, then you are probably in favor of looking at things that can be measured. How is your overall health? What about your cholesterol level and liver function? How about your hormone levels?

Here is an opportunity for both you AND her to be in this together. Go and get your sperm tested, if it hasn't been checked yet. And whilst you're there, get a general checkup done to screen for other health issues that might be brewing.

Anything that comes up in the test results gives us information that we can use to see if additional targeted treatment is needed. This 7 step plan is suitable for all men to follow, and knowing your numbers can give you some markers to retest at the end of the program to see how much change you can measure.

If testing identifies any significant health issues that need to be addressed, I recommend you work in conjunction with an experienced natural fertility practitioner, in addition to working with your medical specialist if your health condition warrants this.

THE SUPER SPERM CHECKLIST

I have developed the below 8-point checklist to determine if there is capacity for your sperm parameters and overall health to be optimized.

If a man experiences one or more of these symptoms, either periodically or ongoing, there is plenty of scope to supercharge his sperm and maximize all his health factors. If you answer YES to one or more of these problems, then there is work to be done to improve your health and optimize your fertility.

Super sperm checklist:

- Fatigue
- Feel flat or low mood (including depression)
- Use reflux or antacid medication
- Use asthma medication
- Losing hair, or starting to go grey
- Aching or pain in the lower back
- Sweat at night in bed
- Digestion isn't great
- Loss of morning erections

While some of these problems may not seem like substantial problems at all, they are all deviations away from optimum health and can be easily improved. In fact, they can become markers to demonstrate not only improved health but also increasing sperm parameters. As the WHO figures provided earlier clearly show, there is a lot of scope for just about every man these days to improve his sperm.

TESTING YOUR SPERM

A comprehensive set of tests will help to reveal any problems. A GP or fertility specialist can order these tests for you to help explore any possibility of your fertility being part of the reason for you not being able to conceive.

CONVENTIONAL TESTS

Physical examination of the testes can help to reveal the presence of any structural abnormalities that are affecting sperm production, such as varicocele. Varicocele is a condition where varicose veins develop around the testes, and as you can imagine, it can have an impact on sperm production. Investigation for varicocele is generally best performed by a urologist, a medical doctor who specialises in male reproductive health.

Hormonal profile: helps to identify problems with the pituitary gland or the testes not producing adequate levels of reproductive hormones.

- **Testosterone**: the total amount of testosterone in the bloodstream, some of which is bound to sex hormone binding globulin (SHBG) and therefore not available for the cells to use.

- **Free testosterone**: the amount of testosterone that is unbound and freely available for cells to use.
- **DHEA**: a steroid hormone that is a precursor to testosterone production. Problems with DHEA levels can cause testosterone levels to be affected, and can point to other potential hormonal imbalances.
- **LH**: luteinising hormone stimulates cells within the testes to produce testosterone.
- **FSH**: follicle-stimulating hormone promotes the growth and maturation of sperm.
- **SHBG**: sex hormone binding globulin attaches to sex hormones such as testosterone and transports them around the bloodstream.

Semen analysis:

- Volume: ideally close to 5ml or more
- Count: ideally 100 million or more
- Motility: ideally 75% or more
- Morphology: ideally 15% or more
- DNA fragmentation

Antisperm antibody: tests for antibodies that fight against a man's sperm. They can potentially be present in the man's own blood, his partner's vaginal fluids, or in the semen itself. Semen can cause an immune reaction in either the man or woman's body.

Serum biochemistry: can give an indication of the overall electrolyte balance within the body and highlight if there are signs the body is struggling to maintain safe levels of acidity/alkalinity.

- **Sodium:** figures in the low range of normal can show that a man may be run down or over-worked

- **Potassium:** can give an indication if there is adequate vegetable intake, and if magnesium status is adequate. If this is very low, it can indicate a problem with kidney function

- **Chloride:** can show if a man is dehydrated or over-worked.

- **Bicarbonate:** can show if there is inadequate deep breathing to clear out all the carbon dioxide. Shallow breathers and those who are stressed and anxious tend to have higher readings.

Liver function: can give us insights into the detoxification potential. Also shows us if there is any liver function impairment related to alcohol or prescription medications, and can also give indications if the body is stressed from over-exercise.

Genetic testing: It is specifically important when investigating fertility to look at the MTHFR gene, which is one of the main genes responsible for methylation.

Methylation problems can increase the risk of miscarriage and can make it more difficult to conceive. Both partners need to be tested, this can help to give an idea of the amount of work that needs to happen in order to get a couple prepared for optimum fertility. If both partners have more than one MTHFR mutation, it can make it much harder to conceive and stay pregnant, with potential babies having very significant MTHFR mutation combinations.

Depending on the results of the MTHFR test, further testing of other genetic mutations is often recommended. It's a good idea to profile the whole genome, rather than just the single MTHFR gene, as there are a number of genetic mutations that play a role in methylation other than the MTHFR gene. There are a large number of companies that offer comprehensive genome profiling. Working with a practitioner who has done in-depth nutrigenomics training on how to use nutrition and natural medicines to reduce the impact of genetic mutations can yield results in improving both partners' health within a short 3-6 month timeframe.

FUNCTIONAL TESTS

The following tests are not part of the conventional approach to investigating male infertility. A natural medicine practitioner, functional medicine doctor or naturopath will be more likely to order these tests for you, and be able to interpret the results.

Plasma zinc: zinc is a crucial nutrient for the production of sperm, and for DNA integrity.

Hair mineral analysis: can give an indication of heavy metal exposure, however the results are not always reliable as it assumes that the heavy metal burden in the body will be excreted in the hair.

Saliva hormone profile: takes a snapshot of the hormonal balance on a particular day and is usually taken in the morning. It tests cortisol, DHEA, testosterone, estrogen and can help to identify if there are problems with hormonal levels at the tissue level. Combined with results from blood tests for hormonal levels it can help to give an understanding not only of overall hormonal levels, but also of availability of hormones at the cellular level.

Urine hormone testing: Specialized testing into hormonal metabolites can give information on specific hormonal imbalances and hormonal processing problems should they exist.

CDSA: complete digestive stool analysis. The health of the digestive system, and bowels in particular, is a vital component of optimal fertility. The bowels and prostate are in very close proximity within the pelvis and so any inflammation or infection present in the bowels can very easily irritate and lead to chronic inflammation of the prostate. Chronic prostatitis can affect male fertility and sometimes can exist without symptoms. Irritation and infection in the bowel can also interfere with normal blood flow and lymph circulation in the pelvis and can affect fertility indirectly. A full assessment of the digestive system can highlight if there are any low-grade bacterial or parasitic infections that might be present and interfering with your fertility potential.

There are some specialist laboratories that provide a complete quantitative assessment of the full microbiome of a person. Assessing the amount of good bacteria, as well as identifying unusual or unhealthy bacteria can help to identify potential digestive imbalances that need to be treated. People with digestive flora imbalances don't always have obvious digestive symptoms, but many have problems such as fatigue, poor concentration, aching lower back or headaches that resolve once the flora imbalance is corrected.

Symptoms that can be related to dysbiosis, you may have only one, or maybe several of these symptoms:

- bloating
- reflux
- diarrhoea
- constipation
- aching joints
- forgetful/memory issues
- headaches
- tired after lunch
- fatigue
- insomnia
- brain fog
- easily distracted

If a stool test shows that you have dysbiosis, working with your health practitioner to improve your digestion will see these issues resolved.

ACTION PLAN

- See your mainstream care provider to get your semen analysis, hormonal investigations and a general health and wellness check.

- Work with a functional medicine or natural medicine practitioner to investigate and address your digestion, mineral status and hormone status.

PART II:

SUPERCHARGE YOUR SPERM

7-STEPS TO BOOST YOUR FERTILITY

Before we officially start on your 7-Step program, have you checked off all the checklist items described in part I of this book? It's important we get as much information as we can about what your starting point is, so that we can see the changes that take place during the program. Ideally you will have done all of the following:

1. You've identified any markers that are relevant to you from the SuperSperm 8 point checklist
2. You've identified any red flags from the Optimal Health checklist
3. You have had your sperm tested
4. You've had a general checkup visit with your GP to assess your general state of health.

Getting these 4 preliminary steps covered will ensure that we make a concerted effort to find any factor coming from your side of the equation that might need to be addressed in order for you to be able to conceive.

The reason you are reading this book, the reason we are talking about this program in the first place, is because something has been missed. One of the reasons you're not pregnant is that something has been overlooked. In all but the rarest cases, there is a reason that you haven't already conceived, and most of these reasons can be corrected.

If nothing has shown up in your test results, or if you're still waiting on your test results to come back - you can still make a start on the program.

What's stopping you from starting today? Nothing? Great - then let's get started.

Step 1: Get your head in the game

Step 2: What should you really be eating?

Step 3: Beware sperm killers

Step 4: Pick up heavy stuff and move it around (exercise for men)

Step 5: Stress management without the woo-woo

Step 6: Natural medicines to supercharge your sperm

Step 7: Staying on track, kicking goals and reaching targets

STEP 1: GET YOUR HEAD IN THE GAME

Ok so I need to reiterate this, in case you didn't start reading right from the beginning (which is totally fine by the way). This book is *not* about sex.

I will not be telling you how to be more manly. Or giving you any advice or critique about your sex life. No talk about your sexuality, your penis, or anyone else's penis for that matter. Just a frank and honest account of what works for my clients in my clinic. I'm a straight shooter, so don't expect anything to be sugar coated and you'll be fine.

So, let's proceed with helping you get your head in the game.

GETTING ON THE SAME PAGE AS YOUR PARTNER

The saying "Men are from Mars, Women are from Venus" too often reflects how couples interact when it comes to preparing to make a baby. But if you can work out how to work together as a team, in a way where you both feel like you're on the same planet, your relationship will become stronger and you'll actually get to enjoy the process together.

For most men, standing by and watching their partner suffer is never high on the list of priorities. The caveman instinct to save the day and be her hero is hardwired into your DNA, lingering close to the surface. But without a to-do list, or a plan of attack to be able to do anything, to be able to make a difference, it can be difficult to even want to engage with the subject at all.

It's time to realise that even though your to-do list is still in the process of being made (don't worry, by the end of this book you will have a to-do list), and your list is not going to be the same as your partner's, you are both on the same journey, and both of you need to make your to-do lists the top priority to strengthen your relationship. The fact that you are soon to be engaged in this process to the same level as her is one of the most awesome parts of the process of building the bond between you both.

Throughout this book, whenever you hear the words "sperm" or "fertility" I want you to imagine millions of strong, healthy sperm who are ready to take on any challenge.

And if you ever think it's too hard, picture your end goal that you're working towards, resting on the couch with your newborn baby sleeping on your chest.

And when you feel like you're going to die if you don't drink alcohol for the next 6 months – know that the amount of physical effort of being pregnant and growing a new person from scratch, and birthing the baby, takes so much more effort than foregoing alcohol for a few months. You'll both be making big sacrifices over the coming months, all for an extremely worthwhile cause of course.

It's not a competition of martyrdom, of who has made the biggest sacrifice, or who is the hardest done by. This process is about lifting the health of both of you so that together as a team you are creating a family that is as happy and healthy as possible from the very start.

"BUT DO I *HAVE* TO DO THAT?"

Let's start with the objections first. Almost everyone has objections; it's hardwired into our DNA to be cautious and critical of change. This book is filled with recommended changes for you to make to all aspects of your life. Some of them you're not going to want to do, some of them you may already be doing. There's a little voice in your head that is going to be second-guessing some of the advice in this book. So, let's have this conversation now before we really get going.

Firstly, something you need to know about me is that I'm a very pragmatic person. As a clinician I am primarily interested in getting results for my clients in the safest, quickest and most effective manner. What that means for you is that I have very little interest in things that don't make a difference. You can show me all the research in the world that demonstrates the positive effect of a particular herb or vitamin has on fertility. However, if I don't see that happen in reality, I don't use it with my patients. Full stop. I don't muck around with things that don't work, and I don't stick with one thing if there is another way of doing it that's more effective, or cheaper, or better. Every piece of advice I put into this book, and into the individualised treatment plans for my clients, represents the best value in terms of the time and effort you'll be investing. I'm more interested in results rather than being a purist of a particular type of approach to the exclusion of others.

I am a natural fertility expert, and people seek my help clinically because of my experience at being able to create a personalized fertility plan and determine the best imple-mentation of that plan for their unique situation. I do have a lot of conversations that turn into negotiations around ways of trimming down the plan:

- "I'm only going to do *this* part of the program, but not *that* part."
- "OK well just tell me what is the bare minimum I have to do. I really don't want to put too much effort into this."
- "What happens if I only do this part, and not that part?"

Yes, these are things that men (and women) really say to me in my clinic every day of the week, so even if you're not thinking these things, other men out there are.

There are many reasons that couples give me for not wanting to participate in their own fertility program:

- "There's nothing wrong with my health; why do I need to do anything?"
- "What are my mates going to say?"

- "I've got a wedding/sports trip/birthday/going away/ celebration/Christmas/new year/vacation to go to so I'll just start all this once that's over."
- "My friends are going out and getting drunk all the time, and their wives got pregnant – why should I have to give up alcohol?"

Well, unfortunately I'm not in charge of the way your body works – there are biological imperatives that we just cannot override. And sometimes life just plain sucks. While some people are out there falling pregnant, first time, every time, others struggle. It's not fair. I get that. Everyone has their own unique body chemistry that we can work to optimize, but not everyone has the same amount of leeway when it comes to alcohol, or sex, drugs and rock 'n' roll.

I can't write you a leave pass from your own body.

Every action we take or don't take has consequences, and I've tried to distill my knowledge and experience into the most effective program that requires the least possible amount of effort and is the most realistic to implement. That said – there's a lot of changes ahead so brace yourself. Get your game face on, and get on with it. Yes, everyone has complaints, yes it's tricky at times, but pretty quickly you will find yourself feeling amazing and full of energy, and possibly having your colleagues and friends asking you about what you've been doing to look so alive. Here is an opportunity for you to really have a massive impact on your own life, and the health potential of your future family. Follow this plan and – as well as super-charging your sperm – you'll be the envy of your friends.

DOING YOUR BIT

Resentment can really build quickly and insidiously in women when they are putting in a whole heap of effort and you're not. On one side of the equation you've got a woman who is really committed to getting herself together: getting her health right, getting her hormones balanced, eating well, exercising, meditating and tracking every single aspect of her menstrual cycle.

Then on the other side of the equation is you. If you're not participating at all in this process, and you're having take away lunches at work, eating dessert at night, having an evening wine or beer, accidentally overindulging in alcohol when on a boys' night out – ask yourself how are your actions in alignment with your goals? It's most likely that your partner has already given up these fun, easy and hedonic pleasures in order for your chances of conceiving to be higher and to improve the health of your as-yet unborn child. However, for some reason, you haven't made changes yet? Every time you indulge, it's a knife in her heart that shows she is on this journey alone. She's thinking that maybe you don't even want a child, or that you don't care about the health of your child. How can you show her that you are committed to this process a

As a fertility expert and natural health practitioner, over the last two decades I have worked with many couples. I have spoken with many men and had a similar conversation with all of them. They approach their appointment with me as a negotiation; that somehow I am the gatekeeper of their health and genetic expression and if I give them a leave pass to continue to do some of the things they are currently doing, that will wipe out the negative effects of what they're doing to their body.

Many people come to my clinic with the mindset that they want to know what is the minimum amount of change and effort they need to put in to be able to get pregnant.

When I talk about this type of attitude and approach with my patients, we have a bit of a play around with the words and we reframe it in a way that makes it easier for them to want to take on board the changes. In fact, many people tell me they don't like how negotiating the bare minimum for their unborn child and the possible health consequences makes them feel selfish and uncaring. There are other ways of describing the type of attitude that doesn't take into account the effects of your actions on another person (and in this case - two people - including your unborn child!).

It doesn't have to be that way - you can choose to be totally on board with this program that *both* of you are taking on. You can happily choose to do more than just the bare minimum, and aim for the best outcome possible.

DO YOU WANT A BARE MINIMUM BABY?

What a concept: bare minimum vs. "this is the best baby I could have possibly made". No one can predict what type of child you will have, what type of health problems your child will face (if any), however the sting of regret is a terrible curse. Speaking as a parent, I know that most parents like to feel they're doing everything they can for their child. Adopting that parent mindset before you even conceive is one of the best things you can do for yourself. You're reading this book which is proof that you're already heading in the right direction, you're already considering making the necessary changes to be in the best shape you can be. To be able to put in place changes in your life that are serving a greater purpose can make the amount of effort required feel substantially less. It doesn't mean you have to be perfect and live your life as a saint, but if you do everything within your power when it comes to your and your partner's health leading up to conception you can stand proud knowing that you did everything you could for your child.

The reality is, every day in clinic I find myself advocating for the health of the unborn child whilst arguing with patients who want to be eating junk food, drinking alcohol, taking illicit drugs, over exercising or not exercising, working in stressful jobs, not getting enough rest, not eating enough nutritious food, and not drinking enough water. All the while, they are grappling with the idea that they have to sacrifice part of their lifestyle a lot sooner than they bargained for in order to reach their fertility potential, and all before the child is even conceived.

Until such time as a couple can hold that space for themselves, my job is to help the potential parents to adopt as many changes as they can that are going to have a positive effect on their unborn child. Prenatal nutrition plays a huge role in the genetic potential and health potential of human beings. It's still a fairly new area of scientific investigation, but the more we look, the more we find that so much of what we consider to be genetic or inevitable when it comes to health is actually partly within our control. Every aspect of unhealthy lifestyle that is investigated is found to have a measurable effect at the other end of the deal.

DON'T BE A VICTIM OF FOMO

One of the things we are going to talk about right here at the start, is your strategy for dealing with FOMO. Fear Of Missing Out. FOMO is a big deal. Usually on weekends and holidays. Special occasions that socially we like to ear-mark with drinking alcohol and eating indulgent unhealthy food.

It's one of the most common discussions I have with my male fertility patients in-clinic. The conversation usually goes a little like this:

Patient: "There's a <special event> coming up - can I <break the program somehow> that day/night/weekend/week?"

Me: "Are you asking to find out if there's a way for you to do this without jeopardizing your progress?"

Patient: "Um, yeah."

Me: "No, there isn't."

Patient: "What about <breaking the program in a reduced or different way>?"

Me: "No."

Patient: "The answer is always going to be no, isn't it?"

Me: "I can't write you a leave pass from your own body. Any deviation from the program will compromise your results. So let's talk about what you're going to say to your friends/colleagues/family members when they want to know why you're not drinking."

Unfortunately many of the ways we have of socialising with our friends, family and work colleagues involves either eating out, or drinking alcohol, or a combination of both. Part of what you're committing to as you implement these 7 steps, is to make the best sperm possible, and in turn, make the best baby possible. I certainly don't want to compromise on either of those outcomes, and I want to support you to be able to successfully complete the program.

Part of what helps people to be successful in making these changes includes having pre-prepared answers to questions they know they will get, and strategies for dealing with the inevitable social situations that will arise over the duration they are on the program.

There is always going to be some event happening in your life to be celebrated. Someone's birthday, maybe even your own birthday, someone getting married, someone going away, your grandmother baked biscuits especially for you, work dinner with prospective clients, catered meetings and conferences. You see the theme here, you catch my drift. There's lots of situations you could find yourself in where you aren't in control of what you're eating, and you may be under pressure/tempted to drink alcohol.

Some men I know are upfront with their reasons for not drinking, and for having dietary changes. They let people know exactly what they're up to:

- We're having trouble getting pregnant, and we are doing a 3 month detox to improve our fertility and improve our chances of getting pregnant.

Other men choose not to be so upfront about the reason for their changes. There are many factors why a man or a couple would want to do this, ultimately your health is your business - not anyone else's and you should only share information about yourself that you feel comfortable disclosing.

Some couples I have worked with are more private with their fertility journey, and so they prefer to use more vague or general reasons like:

- I'm doing a detox.
- I found out I have high cholesterol.
- I'm trying to lose weight.
- I have a new personal trainer and I'm aiming for some big goals.
- I'm on new medication and I've been told I can't drink whilst I'm on it.

Feel free to be creative, and find something that resonates with you, and that feels authentic - afterall you don't necessarily want to be outright lying to people who are close to you and care about you.

You may also need to plan ahead, especially if you're eating out, or at a friend's house. It might involve a phone call or an email to the restaurant ahead of time to check what is on the menu that fits your requirements. Or if you're going to a friend's house for dinner, a phone call or email to your friend outlining your dietary changes and perhaps offer some meal suggestions or offer to bring something to share with others that you can eat too.

The point is that you have a plan, so that you can go into any social situation confident that you'll be able to maintain the integrity of your effort over the coming weeks and months as you implement the steps in this program.

IDEAS FOR REFLECTION:

1. Think about what you are doing to support this journey the both of you are on. Is there anything you could be doing better? Is there anything you'd like to be doing differently? What changes can you make today? What changes can you make this week? Write them down and follow them.

2. Sign up for the email version of this program, delivered to your inbox a few times each week. You will get reminders of where you're up to in the program, the checklists and info you need to get the most out of the program, as well as extra hints and tips. Do this at clarepyers.com/supercharge so that you can be supported in staying motivated for the remainder of the program.

3. How are you demonstrating that you are supportive of her and the fertility journey you are both on? Is it just in your words but not your actions? Is there anything you could be doing better? Is there anything you'd like to be doing differently? What changes can you make today? What changes can you make this week? Write them down and follow them.

4. How do you both feel about talking to friends/family/colleagues about being on this program? Decide on an approach to notifying each group of people about the changes you'll be putting into place over the coming weeks and months.

5. Look at your calendar for the next 3 months. Mark out which social events you will need to navigate and come up with an action plan for getting through each one without drinking alcohol and without deviating from your eating plan. Do you need to contact anyone ahead of time to notify them of your dietary requirements?

ACTION PLAN

- Get your head in the game
- Get yourself together. Make the changes and don't complain
- Bare minimum baby vs. we did everything we could
- Really, you're making these changes for your unborn child
- Life's not fair, play the hand you're dealt

- Don't try to negotiate yourself away from your fertility potential
- Don't be a victim of FOMO

STEP 2: GET YOUR DIET SORTED

Having a clear nutrition plan that is based on tried and tested techniques, and isn't based on the latest fad, is essential if you want to supercharge your swimmers. Every day sees the christening of a new "superfood" only to find out the next day that the superfood isn't so great anymore.

When it comes to eating well - there are a lot of different ideas about what this might look like. The standard Western diet is full of too many grains and other high calorie, low nutrient foods, and doesn't contain enough vegetables, fruits and animal proteins that contain dense nutrient profiles.

In this chapter I'm going to outline specifically what you SHOULD be eating more of in order to optimize your fertility. And just as importantly what you should be AVOIDING so you don't hijack your fertility in the process.

YOU MUST EAT WELL TO OPTIMISE YOUR BABY-MAKING POWERS

Healthy lifestyle, diet and exercise play an important role in fertility. Having a nutritious diet helps to bring hormones back into balance and provides you with all the nutrients you need to optimize your fertility. In many cases of infertility, some nutrients are so depleted that supplementing and targeted diet is required to correct the problem.

When working with couples, I create specific diet plans tailored for individuals. However, there are certain foods everyone needs to avoid due to their negative impact on hormones and fertility; and other foods that are good for all, such as green vegetables. Include green vegetables in equal quantities to the rest of your meal along with coloured vegetables, protein and minerals, as they are all essential for good fertility. Healthy fats deserve a special mention as they are essential for building your hormones, healthy eggs and sperm.

So, let's have a look at what you need to do to take control of your diet.

EATING ORGANIC

Pesticides and other chemicals that make their way into the food we eat have a profound negative effect on your hormonal health. Eating for fertility and hormonal optimization involves eating organic foods and reducing your exposure to pesticides and other hormone disrupting chemicals that are present in the food chain.

Organic foods are grown without the use of harmful pesticides, and don't contain other harmful compounds like BPA in their packaging. Certified organic logos let you know that the product adheres to the strict standards laid out by the regulatory authority that issues the logo.

Eating organic food is especially important when consuming animal products including milk, cheese and yoghurt, as well as flesh. Non-organic foods contain significantly higher quantities of hormone disrupting substances: food crops are sprayed with chemicals, and animals are given antibiotics and other medications that can be found in their milk as well as their flesh. Eating as much organic produce as possible will reduce the total amount of chemicals your body is exposed to, and therefore reduce the extent to which your hormones are being thrown off balance by external factors.

If you can't afford to eat organic, you can grow your own vegetables or purchase locally grown vegetables fresh from a farmers' market where you can ask the farmer in person about their produce and the way it's grown.

YOU NEED ADEQUATE PROTEIN

Protein is the basic building block of the human body, many of us know that protein is mostly what our muscles are made of, you may also know that protein is also what makes a large amount of our connective tissue and internal organs, our hair, skin and nails. Protein also plays a vital role in producing the enzymes that run the thousands of functions in the body, our hormones are also made from protein, and healthy body composition relies on adequate protein intake to support the maintenance of lean body mass. Without adequate protein in the body, we simply do not function anywhere nearly as well as we could.

When we are talking about dietary protein, we are essentially referring to the food sources of nitrogen that provide us with the amino acid building blocks that protein is composed of. There are some amino acids that we are able to produce in the body, and some that we cannot synthesise for ourselves and we must get from our diet. There are 9 essential amino acids that we need to obtain from our diet, ideally on a daily basis. The absolute bare minimum is at least 0.8g protein per kg of body weight. I recommend at least 1.5g protein per kg body weight each day. If you're active and work out, you may do better with 2g protein per kg body weight. For a man who weighs 85kg (187lb) this means aiming for 127g or more of protein each day, up to 170g protein if you are active and work out.

To hit this target, consider the following food portion sizes, and approximately how much protein is in each serve:

1 cup (250ml) whole milk	9g
100g (3.5oz) lean meat or lean fish	20-23g
2 eggs	12g
1 cup (250ml) yoghurt	12g
1 slice of tasty cheese	8g
1 cup protein powder (whey)	27g

Plant based sources of protein are less bioavailable for us than animal proteins, and therefore we need to consume approx 20-30% more protein to ensure that we are still reaching our protein requirements:

1 cup (250ml) almond milk	1g

1 cup (250ml) soy milk	6g
1 cup cooked lentils	18g
100g (3.5oz) tofu	5g
1/2 cup (75g) almonds	15g
1 cup protein powder (rice)	15g

Ideally, it's best to get your protein from whole food sources, which come with a wide range of naturally occurring vitamins, minerals and antioxidants. However I realise it's not always possible to have a "perfect" diet that hits all these targets. In these instances, it's far better to use protein powders to supplement your protein intake, rather than fall short.

If you're reading these figures and feeling overwhelmed, or confused, or feeling like there's no way you'll be able to reach your protein target, I recommend investing in working with a nutritionist or a health practitioner who can guide you through this process. The difference it makes when you get adequate protein in your diet is truly remarkable to experience, and I highly recommend making this a priority. If you are only able to commit to one change (even though I do recommend more than the bare minimum), reaching your protein target is the one to focus on. It's a great place to start when tweaking your nutrition.

YOU NEED SIX HANDFULS PER DAY OF COLOURED VEGETABLES

Vegetables are our primary dietary source of antioxidants, and they are a vital component of a diet of someone who is wanting to improve their health. The reason I measure this in handfuls is that a handful measure is scalable to any person of any size – the size of your hand is relative to your stature and therefore the portion size and overall daily target of vegetable intake is suited to your frame. Generally speaking, six handfuls each day is equivalent to about two heaped dinner plates of vegetables, so it's a fair amount of vegetables. You're not going to get to your target by only having vegetables at your main meal at the end of the day. So, you may need to change things up a bit!

Typical nutrition advice often falls short of what people are actually capable of implementing when it comes to vegetables. The rich phytochemical nutrients present in plants have a wide range of powerful healing properties. Antioxidants help neutralize the effects of the modern day compounds we are exposed to. Most of the world's most powerful anti-cancer and anti-inflammatory compounds are found in plants, particularly those that are strongly coloured. Anti-inflammatory foods are important because of the increased levels of oxidation and inflammation that are usually present when a man has impaired sperm parameters. Anti-inflammatory compounds help to support healthy sperm production in a range of ways, depending on the particular compound - some will help to reduce the effects of oxidative stress, some will improve blood flow and nutrient flow to the genital area, others support healthy sperm production and prevent DNA damage to sperm. Better quality sperm means higher chances of you getting pregnant and having a healthy baby.

Generally speaking, the more potent the colour of a plant, the more potent its phytonutrients are. Getting a large proportion of your dietary fiber intake from leafy vegetables, and a moderate amount from starchy vegetables, with less reliance on grain-based foods such as rice, bread and pasta to fill you up, will lead to a greater sense of health and vitality. Aim to get a rainbow of colour on your plate at each and every meal – including breakfast.

Which brings us to …

EAT LIKE A KING AT BREAKFAST

OMG did I really just say have vegetables for breakfast? Yes – I did. You can have a breakfast frittata or omelette with spinach, sun dried tomatoes, capsicum and olives. You could add some greens to a smoothie. There's no law to say we need to have cereal or toast for breakfast, although thanks to decades of marketing we think that if we miss out on Weet-Bix or Corn Flakes for breakfast that our day is going to be downhill from there. In fact, having a breakfast soup or even having a stir fry or casserole for breakfast helps you to follow the old saying: "Eat like a king at breakfast, a prince at lunch and a poor man at dinner." It provides you with a good serve of nutrients at the start of the day and can help you to get through your day being more effective, more productive and making better decisions.

If you are required to eat out at lunch or for your evening meal it can sometimes be worthwhile to monitor your overall food intake, especially if you're not going to be too active, or not planning on exercising that day. Overeating and gaining weight is not part of what we're trying to achieve here. What we are trying to do is increase your overall intake of nutrients each day by adding vegetables to each meal. Even if you don't have a full meal at breakfast time – which is better suited to those who don't have social constraints over their eating – you can still adjust your thinking a little so that you can plan your nutrient intake.

DITCH SANDWICHES

Relying only on one main meal of the day for the majority of your nutrients is not the way to win at this game. If you're having cereal for breakfast and a sandwich at lunch – even if it's a salad sandwich, you're just not going to hit your target of six vegetables for the day. You're also going to be a long way from being able to reach your minimum amount of protein with the mall amount of meat or cheese that goes into a typical sandwich. Making sure that your lunches are filled with vegetables is the key to reaching your six handfuls of vegetables – this can be a salad, steamed vegetables or some roast vegetables. You can have this large portion of salad or vegetables alongside a robust palmsize or larger serve of fish or meat, with a serve of rice to bulk things up even more if you're needing extra fuel.

SNACKS TO GET YOU OVER THE LINE

Try to get at least three of your six handfuls of vegetables by lunchtime – this could mean having a mid-morning snack of veggie sticks with dip or veggie muffins or frittata for a morning snack. If you're easily reaching your six handfuls of vegetables each day, then you can add in more serves of things like rice and fruit.

Men who are more active will typically need the extra density of calories that come from starchy foods like rice, pasta and sweet potatoes, and usually they have a larger appetite to go along with it. Snacks like rice cakes and crackers can provide a lot of calories in fairly small portions compared to vegetables, which is perfect if you're in an active job, or on days when you're exercising or exerting yourself.

YOU NEED 1 OR 2 PIECES OF FRUIT PER DAY

If you're getting your six handfuls per day of coloured vegetables, you might wonder how on earth you're going to fit in even more food. Fruits contain lots of great health-promoting compounds as well, but they also contain quite a lot of sugar – it's naturally occurring sugar so as long as you're eating the whole fruit it's not a problem, but I want to focus on you getting more bang for your buck when it comes to filling up your belly with healthy food. Generally speaking there are more nutrients in vegetables than there are in fruit, so stick to just one or two pieces each day.

Many fruits contain high amounts of pectins, which help to lubricate and cleanse the digestive system, so if you're visiting the toilet too often then watch your fruit intake. A home remedy for loose bowels is to eat under-ripe bananas – the higher starch content can help to slow down the bowels. If you're noticing things are a little sluggish in that department, go for bananas that are super ripe and have black spots on them, or fruits like apples, pears and plums.

REFINED SUGAR, PRESERVATIVES AND PROCESSED FOODS

Highly processed foods are public enemy number one when it comes to dietary influences on your fertility. Refined sugar and chemical based preservatives are found in just about all processed foods, and almost anything you buy that is in a packet will have some kind of added sugar or chemical on the ingredients list. Say goodbye to sugar and refined foods and you can say goodbye to many troublesome symptoms you are currently experiencing. Some people notice that a large number of health issues disappear altogether with just this step alone. You'll be improving your health and maybe also drop a few unwanted kilos in the process.

HEALTHY FATS ONLY PLEASE

What are healthy fats? Healthy fats are those that contribute to overall health and wellbeing. Plant-based fats including avocado, nuts, coconut oil, seeds and spreads like tahini or almond butter are all good sources of healthy fats.

Animal fats are also good for you in moderation, especially when from organically raised meat. The inflammatory profile of organically raised meat is not as high as meat that is conventionally raised with potential exposure to antibiotics, pesticides and other compounds added to animal feed. Stick primarily to white fleshed animals such as chicken, pork and turkey, and limit red meat intake to no more than two serves per week. Go for low fat cuts if you are hoping to lose a few kilos in this process.

Fish are also an excellent source of protein, and there are some great low-fat fish options that can support weight loss if that is one of your goals.

It's important to note that our oceans are not the clean, pristine environments that they were in the past, with a range of environmental disasters compounding the general levels of toxic contaminants that have found their way into the world's waterways. Eating large predatory fish at the top of the food chain exposes us to higher levels of these chemicals, so the ideal fish to eat are those that are small to medium sized only. Small fish like mackerel and herring are super tasty when they are bought fresh from the market and cooked the same day. If your only experience with sardines is the ones from a can, with or without tomato sauce, you need to reacquaint yourself with this healthy, yummy fish. Do yourself a favor and go to the market and get some fresh sardines, and grab yourself a good recipe.

One of the benefits of eating smaller fish like sardines, anchovies, whitebait, and shellfish is that you get the benefit of eating the entire animal. Generally speaking this means they have a broader and more complete nutrient profile, because you are eating the entire animal including the bones (an excellent source of calcium) and the glands (great for hormonal support). When eating a fish fillet from a larger fish, these same benefits are not available because the bones, glands and organs are usually discarded or re-purposed to other industries.

The only caution with shellfish is that they are a common allergen, and can set off histamine reactions in those who are prone to allergies, and sometimes more severe reactions like anaphylaxis. For many people with sensitive skin (eczema, psoriasis, heat rashes etc.) shellfish can set off inflammation in the body and make skin problems worse. For these reasons, only moderate amounts of shellfish are recommended, and only for those people without skin problems, or without a tendency for allergies.

Stay away from large predatory fish that accumulate heavy metals and toxins (keep servings to a maximum of one serve per month), including:

- tuna
- swordfish
- flake
- orange roughy

Eat only moderate amounts of shellfish (maximum three serves per week) and only if you have no skin problems, including:

- calamari
- mussels
- oysters
- prawns
- lobster

Eat smaller fish that contain less heavy metals and toxins (2-3 serves per week), including:

- herring
- mackerel
- sardines
- anchovies
- white bait

OTHER STUFF

Include avocados, butter, eggs, soaked nuts, sesame seeds or tahini, pumpkin seeds (pepitas), and a moderate amount of animal fats from organic meats, eggs, butter and ghee in your diet.

Cook only with coconut oil or organic ghee. Olive oil is great for drizzling over the top of already cooked food like steamed vegetables. Because it's mono-unsaturated it doesn't remain stable when heated so don't heat it beyond eating temperature to preserve most of the nutritional benefits .

DO YOU NEED TO LOOK MORE CLOSELY AT YOUR DIGESTIVE HEALTH?

Some of the signs associated with poor digestion are: bloating, loose stool, gas, gurgling in the belly, foggy thinking, cold hands and feet, poor circulation, easy bruising, varicose veins, haemorrhoids, heavy menstrual periods in women, and fatigue.

Poor digestion can be caused by:

- irregular eating habits
- eating late at night
- not eating regularly
- overeating
- eating too much cold or raw food
- drinking with meals
- worry
- overwork
- illness
- eating inappropriate foods for your constitution
- stress
- food allergies
- certain medications.

With a weakened digestion, you are not able to effectively absorb all the nutrients in your diet, leading to malnutrition and fatigue. Struggling to digest and process the foods you eat leads to further digestive upset such as abdominal bloating. Without the proper nutrients, your circulatory system and blood vessel integrity can also become weakened – leading to easy bruising, varicose veins and poor circulation. The key to recovery is to strengthen the digestion so that your body can be nourished once again.

FOOD ALLERGIES

It is also important to avoid any foods you are allergic or intolerant to. This reaction is not an anaphylactic-type reaction but rather a reaction that happens in the digestion, usually as a result of increased intestinal permeability (sometimes called "leaky gut"). Certain proteins have made it through your intestine wall and into the bloodstream before they have had a chance to be broken down into an acceptable format. Your body then identifies it as a substance that shouldn't be there and launches an immune response. With repeat exposure this immune response solidifies so that your body reacts on each exposure to that food.

It can be especially worthwhile to test for reactions to common allergens such as wheat, eggs, nuts, gluten and dairy products. This can be done by avoiding all possible sources for at least three weeks, and then reintroducing and checking for re-emergence of symptoms.

However, the fastest and most accurate way to find out which foods your body is sensitive or intolerant to is an IgG food sensitivity test. The IgG food sensitivity test is a blood test that detects antibodies that your body has developed against certain foods. You may have an allergen to foods like corn, eggs, certain nuts or yeast. It is very difficult to ascertain our allergens to these types of foods, as they are hidden in so many processed foods that we eat and we may not know when we are eating them.

Removing foods that you have an IgG reaction to can help to alleviate symptoms associated with exposure. Common symptoms include:

- constipation
- loose bowels/diarrhoea
- abdominal pain/cramping
- bloating
- fatigue
- low mood/fluctuating mood
- skin conditions.

GLUTEN

Gluten has come under a lot of scrutiny in the past few years and has been the subject of many studies and trials. Gluten has not emerged favourably from the majority of these trials and is linked with problems ranging from insomnia and depression through to abnormal sperm results, endometriosis and unexplained infertility.

I recommend that any man or woman wanting to conceive should remove all gluten from their diet. Medicine and science are learning more about gluten and its role in fertility, with new research being regularly published. My clinical observations and recommendations for all my fertility patients to be gluten free are being supported with a growing body of scientific data. There are a number of studies that have found increased pregnancy rates in infertile couples who followed a gluten free diet. Some of the proposed mechanisms include non-celiac gluten sensitivity, and undiagnosed celiac disease. In both these scenarios, the ingestion of gluten containing foods leads to an increase in inflammation in the body that can linger for days, and in some case as long as weeks or months after the exposure to gluten. This inflammation, when chronic, can impair normal reproductive health.

Zinc, selenium, iron, vitamin D, and calcium deficiencies can arise as a result of gluten intake regardless of whether or not you have celiac disease. These nutrients are vital to proper hormonal balance including thyroid function, DNA production, and oxygenation.

One of the most common questions I am asked by patients when we recommend they go gluten-free is, "What can I eat for breakfast?" Gluten-free breakfasts are so wide and varied and can include:

- rice cereal with stewed or sliced pears, cashew nuts and rice or coconut milk
- hot millet/quinoa/amaranth grains (can alternate) porridge
- cranberry flaxseed granola
- eggs with bacon and steamed greens
- steamed or pan fried fish with fresh herbs
- omelette
- protein pancakes with maple syrup
- fruit and yoghurt
- soup

- leftovers

FERTILITY KILLERS

By now you might be starting to imagine yourself putting 100% effort into hitting your targets, making sure you're getting plenty of vegetables, eating the right types of protein and getting your breakfast right.

The next step is to make sure you're not inadvertently hijacking your hormones and the sperm production process, so let's avoid you eating these foods:

Avoid/reduce processed food and sugar

These foods will often contain ingredients that can negatively impact your fertility such as soy or gluten or trans fats. They often contain additives, chemicals and added sugar that can also hijack your hormones.

Avoid soy-based foods

Soy has a negative impact on thyroid function - it blocks the uptake of iodine into the thyroid gland and can lead to decreased levels of thyroid hormone and increased levels of thyroid hormone antibodies.

Avoid all alcohol

Alcohol consumption kills sperm in multiple ways - reducing overall numbers of sperm, making them swim slower and more likely to be the wrong shape. Alcohol also lowers testosterone levels, increases estrogen levels and makes your overall reproductive hormone levels imbalanced.

Avoid coffee – even 1 cup per day can create hormone imbalance

Your one cup of coffee each day may feel insignificant in terms of your overall health, but it can increase your risk of miscarriage. The goal of this program is to have a baby - not just to get pregnant. We want you to have a successful pregnancy.

Avoid soy foods – they can create hormone imbalance

Soy is a common food that is generally regarded as a health food. However - this is not the case, it can elevate estrogen levels in your body which will reduce your sperm production. It also blocks the normal functioning of the thyroid gland - this can increase your chances of weight gain and general imbalance within your endocrine (hormonal) system. It's in lots of packaged foods - check your labels and you'll be surprised!

Avoid sugary drinks and soft drinks/fizzy drinks

Sugary drinks can wreak havoc with your blood sugar levels especially when consumed on an empty stomach. Many soft drinks in addition to large amounts of sugar, also contain colours and additives that can be inflammatory and worsen your overall health as well as your hormonal balance.

Avoid refined sugar and artificial sugars

Artificial sugars are chemical compounds that have unwanted effects on the body including on your cognitive function and your hormonal balance. Some artificial sweeteners break down into toxic by-products like formaldehyde. Wholefood based sweeteners such as honey and maple syrup are better alternatives.

Avoid fat-free foods

Unless you're going for a natural fat-free food like a carrot, or an apple, odds are you're looking at a food that is highly processed and high in sugar, and likely contains numerous additives. Go for whole foods, and don't be afraid of naturally occurring fats if you're eating a healthy diet of veggies, fruit, meat, eggs, fish.

Avoid trans fats found in processed and fried foods

Fat is not bad for you - the 80s did a lot of damage to our collective psyche. However, TRANS FAT is very bad. It is found in almost all processed and fried foods. Foods like margarine are very high in trans fat - and they should not be consumed by anyone. Trans fats are the dangerous fats that contribute to inflammation and heart disease risk. Avoid them at all costs

Avoid refined carbohydrates like white bread, cakes and biscuits

Grain based foods can create inflammatory responses in a lot of people, especially when they are in the form of highly processed foods such as white bread, cakes and biscuits. Lectins and anti-nutrients like phytates are present in wheat flour and can reduce your absorption of all other nutrients from your diet. Wheat crops are also heavily sprayed with pesticides so unless you're eating foods made from organic wheat flour, then you're also getting a large dose of pesticide which is known to kill off your gut bacteria. Double whammy for your gut.

Avoid Commercial White Bread

All commercial wheat flour in Australia has added synthetic folic acid - this type of folate is added to support the prevention of neural tube defects, which is an important reason to take folate. However the toxic form of folate - folic acid - can be carcinogenic and promote infertility and this is the form that is in commercially sold white bread. It's best to avoid commercial white bread for this reason, and go for an organic, sourdough bread from your local bakery instead. Get the safe form of folate from your multivitamin. More on supplements in chapter 11.

Avoid any other highly processed foods

Generally high in calories, and contain multiple food additives that have negative effects on your body. They are usually not health promoting foods.

Avoid large deep-water fish

Large, deep-water fish are fish like tuna, shark (flake), whale, swordfish. They contain large quantities of mercury and other dangerous compounds that bioaccumulate in the environment. Weight for weight, smaller fish contain a much smaller percentage of contaminants compared to these larger fish. Go for smaller fish like salmon, whitebait, sardines, mackerel, shellfish, barramundi etc.

FERTILITY SUPERFOODS

Eggs – farm fresh free range with dark orange/yellow yolks

Nuts and Seeds – especially almonds, walnuts , flax seeds, chia seeds, pumpkin seeds, sesame seeds, sunflower seeds, hemp seeds.

Brazil nuts – highest food source of selenium, supports testosterone. **Pumpkin seeds** – zinc.

Fish and shellfish – eat mostly cold water fish (like Alaskan salmon and cod), avoid large deep water fish (like tuna steaks and swordfish) because of the potential for high mercury levels

Grass-fed organic meats have higher levels of nutrients, and less chemical exposure

Liver is exceptionally nutrient dense

Dark leafy green vegetables – especially spinach, broccoli, kale and collards **Colourful vegetables** – eat a wide variety daily that are in season

Fruit – eat ripe and raw; fruits highest in antioxidants are prunes, pomegranates, raisins, blueberries and strawberries

Goji Berries – packed with antioxidants

Raw cacao nibs – magnesium, iron and potassium

DO YOU NEED TO LOSE A FEW KILOS?

Earlier in the book we talked about the link between men who are overweight or obese having a lower sperm count, lower sperm motility, lower normal morphology (shape), increased DNA fragmentation, lower testosterone levels and higher estrogen levels. Basically - stuff that lowers your ability to make an amazing baby.

Losing weight is a great goal to have if you want to improve your fertility and improve the quality of sperm that will go towards making your child.

For men, the best way to lose a few kilos and embark on a healthy eating program to lose body fat is to follow a wholefood based ketogenic diet for a period of 6-8 weeks. A ketogenic diet consists primarily of eating coloured vegetables, contains moderate amounts of proteins, moderate amounts of healthy fats and is low in starchy carbohydrates.

This technique is useful in the short-medium term by supporting fat loss, while supporting the body to maintain muscle mass. When carbohydrate intake is restricted, the body burns fat for fuel instead. You are also avoiding many packaged and processed foods, thereby reducing your overall inflammatory load in your body. Provided that dietary intake of calories is not excessive, the body can then begin to access fat stores for fuel. This approach to weight loss focuses on nutrient dense foods that support fat burning and also help to flood your body with nutrients, and remineralise and detoxify your entire body.

Stage 1: Quick weight loss – 6-8 weeks

3 palm-sized serves of meat or fish each day

6 handfuls of non-starchy vegetables each day

1 handful of non-starchy fruit each day

1-2 tablespoons of healthy fats each day

2 optional protein snacks each day

Avoid starchy foods such as potato, sweet potato, corn, banana, mango, rice, wheat, bread, pasta, oats and barley.

Stage 2: Continued weight loss

Add some non-gluten starches back into your diet one or two days a week initially; this is best timed after exercise and helps to transition you back to a longer term eating pattern that you'll hopefully be able to maintain. It also allows you to assess the effects of starchy foods and high GI foods on your weight, energy levels and mood in a controlled way. Some people find they do really well with two servings of rice each week, but if they add in three or four servings that's when they start to feel sluggish, start to regain weight or get a bit grumpy.

Some people will find that even one serving of bread or pasta can have them literally gain 1-2kg overnight, and it takes a few days for the weight to fall off again. For these people I recommend to stay off gluten for a longer period of time, and then go for a smaller serve, or for a low gluten variety like spelt. Having certified organic products can also reduce the level of reactivity; sometimes the reactions to gluten are magnified by the presence of glyphosate "Roundup TM" which is a pesticide used widely in the farming of wheat particularly in Australia and the USA.

If you gain 1-2kg overnight, this can be a sign of food intolerances. You can learn more about how to overcome food intolerances in my online course, or by working with an experienced practitioner who can help you to identify and work through this health issue.

Find out what your body wants and needs

The important thing is to use the transition period from stage 1 to stage 2 as a way to learn a bit more about your unique biochemistry. Scientific studies can only tell us about averages and generalizations, and every study has statistical outliers who have results that are different from the others. Find out what your body wants and needs, learn how to listen to those messages and you will start to discover that there are helpful signposts along the way that help to guide you towards healthier eating that suits you. Experiment a little, but be open to hearing the messages from your body – if your weight goes up, you notice fluid retention or you get grumpy, it's a sign that you were previously in balance but now you're not.

Forget the concept of "If this food is healthy how could it be bad for me?" We are all unique individuals and there is no one food that is guaranteed to be good for everyone.

NO SHORTCUTS

Eating the right foods is one of the most important things that will dictate your level of success on this program. It's not just about how much you weigh, it's important for men with a naturally fast metabolism to watch what they eat too. The chemistry of what the compounds in our food do to our bodies is of vital importance when it comes to improving your overall health, reaching optimal hormonal balance and supporting great sperm production.

There are no shortcuts here. You have to do the work. Eat natural whole foods that are provided to us by nature, eat the least amount of processed food possible, and you will see positive changes in your mood, energy levels and more within just a few short weeks.

Spend this week getting the hang of this new way of eating. Next week we are going to make sure you are avoiding the most common things that are going to hamper your fertility efforts - the Sperm Killers Checklist.

ACTION PLAN

1. Set aside an hour or two to go through all the items in your cupboards and your refrigerator and freezer. Check the labels. Do they contain soy? Wheat or other gluten? Do they contain additives like MSG (flavor enhancer 621, 631 etc). If so - throw them out. Do you have margarine in the fridge? Throw it out too.

2. Find some local suppliers for good quality food products: organic butcher, sourdough bakery products, organic fruits and vegetables, organic dairy products. Focus on sourcing good quality ingredients, so that you can be sure you're getting the nutrients you need from the food you're eating.

3. Increase your intake of fruit and vegetables.

4. Ensure you're hitting your protein target on a daily basis. 1.5g protein per kg body weight, up to 2g protein per kg body weight if you are active and work out.

5. Keep an eye out for food intolerances or food allergies. Work with a practitioner or complete my online Freedom From Food Intolerance Workshop to know what you should do about this.

STEP 3: BEWARE SPERM KILLERS

Our homes, our food and our workplaces are filled with compounds that are toxic, hormone-disrupting chemicals that are proven time and time again to damage sperm, affect DNA replication and interfere with hormone levels. Some of them are known as xenoestrogens, meaning they act like estrogen in the body. For men, this can lead to the debilitating condition known as "man-boobs". We recommend you avoid these chemicals at all costs and change to products that are safe, natural, and don't lead to you needing to purchase a man-bra.

CHEMICALS TO WATCH OUT FOR

The following are chemicals that you should watch out for – these can be present in anything from toothpaste, shampoo, skin moisturiser and hand soap through to household cleaning products including clothes washing detergent, dishwashing liquid and surface cleaners.

There are also certain compounds including plastics and treated wood products that contain potent xenoestrogens that can interfere with the way your hormones function within the body.

Formaldehyde: present in MDF (medium density fibre-board) and furniture such as drawers, cabinets etc. made from this wood product. Also look out in personal care and products for ingredients such as DMDM hydantoin, diazolidinyl urea and quaternium 15.

Phosphates: present in many cleaning products including automatic dishwasher tablets, dishwashing liquid, laundry liquid. Watch out for chemical names like sodium tripolyphosphate. Go for products that state Phosphate Free on the label.

PBDEs: polybrominated diphenyl ethers are used as flame retardants in carpets, upholstered furniture, mattresses (especially those manufactured prior to 2005), and electronics manufactured prior to 2014.

Sodium lauryl sulphate: present as a sud-forming agent in shampoo, soap and washing detergent.

Triclosan: present in antibacterial cleaning products such as soap and hand rubs. Go for alcohol-based hand rubs instead, or soap without added ingredients.

2-Butoxyethanol: present in window cleaners and kitchen cleaning products.

Bisphenol A (BPA) and phthalates: present in shopping receipts, softened plastics like the plastic used in raincoats and backpacks, plastic drink bottles and food containers, the lining of food cans, and perfumed products (especially when "fragrance" is listed) such as air fresheners, toilet paper, perfume and aftershave.

OTHER THINGS TO LOOK OUT FOR

- The enzymes required for sperm production are very sensitive to heat. The reason that the testicles hang away from the body is that it's about 4 degrees cooler than normal body temperature. In order to ensure good sperm health:

  - Keep laptops away from your lap and turn off the Wi-Fi if you have to use them on your lap. Lap trays can be purchased which can help to reduce the heat transferred to your body.

  - Take your mobile phone out of your pocket. Keep it away from your body, or at the very least keep it in your chest pocket, or your back pocket away from your groin.

  - Avoid spas, saunas and hot tubs, to ensure your sperm are not subjected to heat that may be damaging.

  - Ensure your underwear are loose fitting and not too tight. Allowing for adequate ventilation and circulation helps to keep the scrotum cool and functioning optimally.

  - Avoid riding a pushbike, instead walking or running are better forms of exercise that don't put pressure onto the groin.

MOBILE PHONES

I'm putting it here twice, because it deserves to be here twice. Mobile phones have been shown to kill sperm. When a person has a phone in direct contact with their body, they are exceeding the as-tested guidelines for safe exposure to RF radiation. A study performed in 2014 showed that significant changes to progressive motility (the number of sperm swimming in the right direction) and DNA fragmentation in sperm that were exposed to mobile phone radiation for 5 hours. The changes in DNA fragmentation were apparent in as little as 1 hour of exposure to mobile phone radiation. The level of exposure to mobile phone radiation is at its highest as your phone rings with an incoming call, and during times when you are in low reception areas.

The long and short of it is - if you want to pass on your genetic material at its best, without as few mutations as possible - get your mobile phone out of your pants pocket and away from your genitals!

ABSTINENCE

"Keep the pipes clean." Ejaculating daily helps the turnover of sperm and is thought to promote better morphology. A healthy man can replenish sperm each day, and there is no need to save up sperm for days at a time. Regular intercourse is also thought to improve the woman's immune response to the sperm and she is therefore less likely to have antibodies to the sperm.

SMOKING

You need to stop smoking. Studies prove that men who smoke have lower numbers of sperm and have lower motility (they swim slowly or not at all). Fertility is significantly impaired if either the male or the female partner is a smoker. Smokers require nearly twice the number of IVF attempts as non-smokers. Clinically I have seen sperm antibodies occur much more commonly in men who are smokers, than in men who don't smoke.

UNNECESSARY PRESCRIPTION MEDICATIONS

Reduce or eliminate unnecessary prescription and non-prescription medications. Many people are on medications for necessary reasons – diabetics take insulin, people with Hashimoto's take thyroxine, people with asthma take inhaled steroids. It's important for people to stay on these medications to keep their condition under control.

However there are many people who take medications unnecessarily. Painkillers are a commonly overused medication. Examples include:

- Drinking too much alcohol (which is bad for sperm anyway) then taking paracetamol for the hangover the next day.

- Eat a diet filled with processed food and minimal fresh food and then take antacid medication for reflux.

- Don't drink water or exercise or eat enough fibrous vegetables and then take a laxative for constipation.

I have many conversations with patients every week to help them to identify which medications they may be able to safely discontinue. We then develop a plan and implement it in conjunction with their GP or prescribing physician. The original issue for which your medication was prescribed may already be resolved, or could be easily addressed by the very changes you are undertaking in this program. I do not recommend you stop taking medication without first speaking to your doctor. I do recommend regularly revisiting the list of medications you are on to see if they are still appropriate for you, and discussing alternatives with your health care provider.

DON'T UNDERESTIMATE THESE KILLERS

Whilst this is only a short chapter, and it may seem like there are only a handful of things you need to watch out for, these sperm killers are one of the biggest things to watch out for in your Sperm Supercharge Program. Some of these factors are so significant they can literally reduce your numbers of healthy sperm to almost zero. Take the time to go through each one of these carefully and assess the ways in which you can avoid them in your daily life.

ACTION PLAN

1. Check all your household cleaning products. Do they have "phosphate free" written on the label? Do they contain poison warnings? Look to change over your cleaning products and personal care products to safe brands that don't contain hormone disrupting chemicals.

2. Take your mobile phone out of your pants pocket. Start a new habit of putting it somewhere else - preferably away from your body entirely. Back pocket and shirt pocket are a compromise - you are still exposed to the radiation but the effects on your sperm production is reduced.

3. Speak to your doctor about reviewing your medications. Are there any that can be reduced or removed? Discuss a plan with a natural medicine practitioner to reduce your reliance on painkillers and medications like antacids.

STEP 4: PICK UP HEAVY STUFF AND MOVE IT AROUND (EXERCISE FOR MEN)

R egular exercise is an important component of a healthy lifestyle. It's easy for it to slip through the cracks for some men. At the end of a busy day or busy week, your best intentions to exercise may have fallen by the wayside and are replaced with late nights at work, social commitments, fatigue or lack of motivation.

As you proceed through the steps in this program, we want to make exercise a priority. By now you've already been eating differently, and hopefully you are starting to feel changes in your energy levels, sleep, mood and motivation. Let's put that extra energy to good use by getting your body and mind into a good exercise routine.

In addition to supporting male hormonal balance, the best exercise program should also create a sense of achievement, as well as meeting the inner desire for caveman chest beating.

AN EXERCISE PROGRAM TO SUPPORT FERTILITY

An exercise program that will support male fertility and male hormone levels – primarily testosterone – needs to be targeted to each individual in order to get the best results. Generally speaking however, exercising and having intentional movement on most days of the week and moving more than you're not is the key to supporting optimum fertility in men.

The way that a man exercises in order to optimize his hormone levels will be very different from the way a woman needs to exercise in order to balance her hormone levels. So bear in mind that unfortunately in this part of the program you and your partner won't be doing the same activities in the same way. The exercise that women need to balance their estrogen and progesterone levels is different and needs to change according to the different phases of their menstrual cycle.

Overall, an exercise program that supports optimum male fertility is one that has an endurance focus. Building endurance will help a man to become strong and will support healthy testosterone levels. With an exercise program that focuses on endurance, the general benefits include improved energy levels and mood and a boosted immune system, and it will not be overly stressful and counteract the benefits of muscle building and hormone balancing.

I'm going to outline here a general exercise program that supports good hormonal balance, improves your testosterone levels, improves your stress resilience, and your overall health and vitality.

If you have a specific medical condition, or injuries, I recommend you work with a qualified exercise physiologist or another exercise specialist who is experienced with prescribing exercise for people with complicated health is-sues.

ENDURANCE PROGRAM

Weight training will boost and support hormone levels, and increase your testosterone levels. Body weight training is also great, including squats, lunges, push-ups and tricep dips. As a general rule, for building muscle and supporting testosterone levels, weights should be heavy. For building endurance, weights should be moderate.

To boost testosterone = 1-8 reps, heavy weight

To build endurance = 15-20 reps, moderate weight.

To boost testosterone levels, the weight that you are lift-ing should be so heavy that you reach "positive failure" in 8 reps or less i.e. you can't physically lift it one more time. As you get stronger, you'll need to increase your weight to keep in this low rep range. This is a good approach for men who need to boost testosterone levels, and it's good to limit this type of workout to once or twice a week only.

In an endurance program, the muscles are spending longer periods of time under strain. This strengthens them but not to the point of exhaustion, and in this way it helps to keep stress hormones at a moderate level, while support-ing healthy testosterone levels. You should not exercise to failure in this exercise approach. Instead, you should finish up feeling like you still have more reps in the tank, and fin-ish the session feeling like you could go longer if you had to. This type of workout is better suited to a man who has a stressful job, who works long hours, or who is experiencing a lot of stress.

The amount of stress you are under in your daily life plays a big role in dictating the type of exercise that is going to benefit you the most. If you don't have enough active and passive recovery built into your life - e.g. leisure, rest, relaxation, meditation, massage, stretching etc., then the benefits of a high stress workout can be lost and can even become detrimental to your efforts. We don't want your exercise program to create more stress than your body can tolerate, even if it helps to increase your testosterone levels.

If you've never lifted weights before - consider working with a personal trainer or someone who can show you the ropes. Working with a trainer gives you the confidence that you know what to do, you can be confident you're getting a good workout and you are less likely to injure yourself.

If you've experienced injury, or are dealing with health challenges, consider working with an exercise physiologist. They have completed university level qualification in prescribing exercise to support health recovery and rehabilitation from injury. They can develop and oversee your program to ensure it's best suited to your requirements.

CARDIO PROGRAM

The best form of cardio training for men is high intensity interval training (HIIT), and you can add it into your other workouts.

High intensity interval training involves periods of intense, short bursts of activity usually between 8-30 seconds, followed by a longer period of recovery activity like walking for 20-60 seconds (sometimes longer).

An example: sprint for 10 seconds, and then walk back to where you started. Then repeat this 3-5 times, up to 10 times if you are already very fit.

Another example is riding on an exercise bike - and getting your RPM above 100 and keeping it there for 20 seconds, and then lowering the RPM down to 60-70 RPM for 60 seconds. Adjust the resistance on the bike to increase the challenge and effort. Repeat up to 10 times.

High intensity interval training doesn't need to be done for a long period of time; at least 4 minutes a couple of times a week is all you need to reap the benefits. In fact, overdoing it can lead to detrimental effects and can result in over training and a negative effect on your health. More than three sessions each week of HIIT can quickly cause damage to your metabolism and hormone balance due to overtraining. Doing HIIT sessions that are long in duration can also damage your metabolism and hormonal balance. This means it's going to lower your testosterone levels and impair your baby making prowess. HIIT training is like the icing on the cake; you need a solid foundation of strength and endurance in order to get the benefits of it and to protect yourself from its potential negative effects.

REST

Active and passive rest days are crucial to the success of any exercise program. Muscle repair occurs only with proper complete rest and proper nutrition.

Counteracting the effects of external emotional stress is vital – whether it's work or home life that's causing stress. However, exercise is also a form of stress on the body; that's what causes muscle fatigue and pain after a weights session. Stress is what causes your mind to want to stop running before you reach your destination. Exercise works to reduce the impact of external emotional stress on our body but to do that, the body requires quality rest time between sessions. Rest days are just as crucial as the days where you are training.

Rest days are where the magic happens. The types of activities you do should be useful in stimulating circulation and blood flow to your muscles in a gentle way to help remove toxins and lactic acid build up. You also want it to stimulate lymphatic flow to further enhance the benefits of exercise by keeping your lymphatic system flowing and able to cleanse the body more effectively.

On active rest days you are doing the restful and recovering activity yourself. Activities such as yoga, stretching and Pilates help the body to assimilate the benefits of exercise and help to promote the continued effects of exercise not only on building muscle mass but also mitigating the temporary stressful effects that exercise can have on the body.

On passive rest days, someone else is doing the rest and recovery for you. Passive rest days include activities such as going for a massage or going for a salt float therapy session.

The amount of rest and recovery you need is going to depend on what the rest of your life is like. If you have a busy life with a lot of stress then getting adequate R&R can be the difference between reaching your health goals or not. And if you're reading this book then one of your main health goals is likely to be improving your health and your overall state of nutrition in order to prepare for becoming a parent.

HOW TO GAUGE THE INTENSITY OF YOUR WORKOUT

It's important for you to get the intensity of your workout right. We want you to put effort in - if you are doing a cardio workout, your heart rate and breathing should be elevated to the point where you can *just* hold a conversation. If you can't do that - back off on the intensity. If you can breathe so freely that you can sing whilst you're working out - you need to step it up.

Pay attention to your recovery from your workouts as well. If you finish a workout so exhausted that you need to go to bed - you've probably overdone it. If you finish your workout feeling like you've done a workout but overall you feel energised and feel the benefits of feel-good compounds like endorphins - then you've probably hit the nail on the head.

WATCH OUT FOR THESE COMMON MISTAKES

It's natural to want to put your best efforts in when it comes to exercise. There's lots of stereotypes for you to live up to regarding machoness, manliness, and your ability to lift heavy weights, or be able to run a marathon.

We don't want to jeopardize the results you've already made so far, and remember you're not trying to get into the Olympics, we want to support hormonal balance and optimize your health. Sometimes super fit people have gone beyond that point of balance - so we aren't aiming for you to be the fittest man you know.

Here are some common mistakes that men can make when undertaking a new exercise program.

- Go from no exercise to smashing yourself 6-7 days per week
- Doing an exercise program that adds more stress to the body than it removes
- Getting the intensity of your exercise program wrong
- "No Pain, No Gain" mantra can lead to injury
- Not getting enough rest in between sessions
- Going to the gym too often
- Incorrect technique with lifting weights can lead to injury

SIGNS YOU'RE GETTING IT WRONG

You may already have an exercise program that you've been following for a while, or you may be just starting out now. No matter what your starting point is, it's important to listen to what your body is telling you.

Here are some signs that you are possibly pushing your exercise program too far for your body to be able to deal with:

- Getting sick
- Getting run down
- Getting injured
- Exhausted rather than energised from your workouts
- Not putting on muscle as you would expect

ACTION PLAN

1. Work with a personal trainer or exercise physiologist to develop a custom exercise program for you that supports your hormonal health. Or join a gym like F45 or Crossfit.

2. Make sure you have a balance of cardio workouts, strength and endurance workouts to balance your exercise program. Take into account the amount of stress you experience in your life to guide your balance of strength and endurance focused weight lifting sessions.

3. Factor in adequate rest and recovery into your program to ensure you don't hijack your results.

4. Make changes before you get injured, seek professional guidance to help you change your workout if you are getting injured, run down or sick.

STEP 5: STRESS MANAGEMENT WITHOUT THE WOO WOO

STRESS AND YOUR PHYSICAL HEALTH AND WELLBEING

Natural medicine puts a heavy emphasis on our emotions as a key driver of physical health and wellbeing. This is almost always the case when it comes to internal medicine and even more so when dealing specifically with fertility.

Stress takes the cake when it comes to hormonal hijacking. Hormones go about their usual business except when your life is in danger – and then all resources are focused on staying alive. Adrenaline, the fight or flight response, sets you up for a hormonal profile that shuts down reproduction in favour of "survival mode".

Fertility treatment – whether by trying naturally or with assisted reproductive technologies – can be an emotionally trying experience on its own before adding the pressures of becoming/being a parent, maintaining a social life and having a career. Today's lifestyle is incredibly stressful, and with the stress that is placed on people today, it's not surprising that fertility issues are increasing. By supporting emotional resilience and reducing the effects of stress on the body, you can go a long way towards improving your emotional, reproductive and general health.

There are many benefits to reducing your stress levels and reversing the effects of burnout. You'll have better concentration and mental performance at work, you'll sleep better, and you'll feel more in control of yourself day-to-day. And it doesn't need to take longer than 10 minutes a day. Anything that reminds your body and mind that your life is not in danger, that you're not about to die, is beneficial. Anything that helps you forget about your troubles will help to reduce your adrenaline levels and allow the space for your hormones to do the right thing. Things you can do to counteract stress include:

- go on a holiday
- learn to meditate
- take up yoga
- get acupuncture or a massage
- take your shoes off and go for a walk along the beach or in a park.

WHEN STRESS BECOMES NORMAL

All emotions, no matter how subtle or strong, have effects that span throughout all layers of a person, including the physical body. Many people today are living under a constant state of stress and may be so accustomed to stress that it is no longer possible to recognise their own stress levels. Some common emotional patterns that can become habitual include worry, overachieving, perfectionism, negative inner dialogue, fear, anxiety, frustration, anger, resentment, overwhelm and melancholy. Every one of these emotional patterns will have a physiological effect. The constant presence of particular neurotransmitters and stress hormones will provide constant stimulation to the whole body.

These emotional patterns are normal, but like all emotions, should come and go and not remain as the dominant way of interacting with yourself and the world. When your physiology becomes familiar with these emotional patterns and gets used to stress hormones circulating in the body, this can become the new homeostatic place that your body and mind will try to maintain. This creates an environment in your body that is very similar to those who have experienced multiple traumas during their formative developmental years. For these people with constant high levels of stress, the mind believes that a stressed state is a natural and safe way to be. The body continues to take its cues from the mind about how the physiology should be, and in response to a stressed mind, a physiological stress response ensues. Constant stress, whether from external circumstances – you ARE actually being chased by a white tiger – or from internal emotional stress patterns that don't switch off, is a big part of what determines your physiology and your hormonal patterns.

If stress hormones are activated and running through the body for long periods of time, in order to keep that set point and feel normal it becomes necessary for stressed people to do things that exhilarate, push, tire, challenge, excite, demand, test and stress the body. Continuing to promote the stress response might satisfy the mind but it continues to push the body in a way that it was not designed for. This aspect of our physiology is there to be used in times of danger, or in the hunt for prey, but with periods of rest, relaxation and reflection in between. Continuing to live in a way that places large demands on your body has negative fertility consequences for both men and women.

If living a stressful existence in the modern world was enough to take a toll on your fertility, add in the stress caused by months or years of trying to conceive unsuccessfully and before you know it, there is stress coming at both the man and woman from all angles. The stress, panic and upset you haven't yet been able to conceive a child unfortunately further reduces your chances of falling pregnant. Stress is such a cruel, double-edged sword.

REDUCING STRESS

Taking steps to reduce stress and embrace a calm inner landscape can be a tough challenge. Spending time each day to relax and reflect is important – this is more than just "switching off" in front of the television, but rather spending deliberate effort to calm your body and mind. For some people, activities like yoga and meditation are useful. For others, a gym session, running or swimming helps. Doing things each day that you enjoy and that make you happy is also important. Stress management doesn't have to involve sitting in locust pose singing Kumbaya.

Most importantly, you will need to retrain your mind to a new set point, to a calmer and more relaxed way of being. Establishing a reference point for your emotional patterns that is closer to neutral allows your mind to stay more connected, leaving you feeling more centred and level headed. This reference point for your emotional patterns also gives your physiology a chance to establish a new point of reference, and lays the foundation for you to alter your health. When it comes to your state of mind, knowing exactly where neutral is – where zero is – gives you the confidence to express your emotions more freely, as and when you experience them, and be able to let go of them and come back to yourself afterwards.

Having a neutral emotional state might feel odd at first, and your body and mind may go through an initial withdrawal period as you adjust to different levels of hormones and neurotransmitters in your body. As your body adjusts and your mind adjusts, you should begin to feel a greater sense of clarity, feel more grounded, and less hurried inside. This process can take time. For some it is as quick as a few weeks, for others it can take months or years to retrain the mind and body into the new reference point.

KEEP IT SIMPLE

If you're dealing with big problems, it can help to break it down into smaller steps, more manageable pieces. This can help your mind to get out of the feeling of overwhelm - which can be paralysing - and get you into an action oriented mindset.

Ask yourself - what smaller steps are going to help me deal with this problem successfully? What can I do today? What can I do this week? Small things can make a big difference.

CREATE POSITIVE MOMENTS

Make as many positive moments as you can in your day. John Gottman is a relationship researcher, he promotes the idea of positive sentiment override. The ratio of your positive:negative thoughts and experiences can dictate how well you and your relationship will survive a stressful time. A ratio of 5:1, where there are 5 times as many positives as negatives, is predictive of your relationship stability to within 97% accuracy.

MEDITATION

A lot of men roll their eyes at me, or stare at me in disbelief when I mention the word Meditation.

Meditation doesn't have to involve sitting with your legs crossed whilst wearing a monk outfit. Not all meditation involves sitting with your eyes closed and trying not to think about anything.

The benefits of meditation on improving your overall health, counteracting the effects of stress, reducing inflammation and balancing your hormones have only recently been uncovered by modern science. Ancient cultures and traditions that incorporate meditation have known for a long time about the benefits of a daily meditation or process of reflection.

You don't need to meditate for hours every day in order to get the benefits. However, there is a funny saying, you should meditate for 20 minutes per day. If you are busy, then you should meditate for an hour every day. Meaning that, the busier your life, the more you need it, and the higher priority it should be.

There are many different ways of meditating. Some people find using an app or listening to audio recordings with guided meditations is well suited to them.

Other people find self hypnosis, or listening to a hypnosis CD is better suited to the way that their mind works.

There are many people and organizations that run meditation classes, some are designed as a course, others are designed as drop-in classes that you can attend anytime.

ACTION PLAN

1. Try out different ways of meditation. Find a way that suits you, and that you can commit to. 10 minutes a day is all it takes.

2. Plan regular activities into your calendar that mitigate the effects of stress in your life. The more stress you experience in your life, or the more busy you are, the higher priority this needs to be, and the more stress relieving activities you need to schedule into your diary.

STEP 6: NATURAL MEDICINES TO SUPERCHARGE YOUR SPERM

N atural medicines are very potent, and when you take the right supplements for you, they can work wonders and make it four times more likely you will conceive. However, knowing which ones are right for you is important, it's vital to avoid the natural medicines that are likely to be detrimental for you, as well as focusing on the ones that will benefit you.

Knowing which supplements are going to give you bang for your buck is important so you're not wasting hundreds of dollars each month on products you don't need, or which might be harming you. Avoid guesswork at all costs and only follow trusted advice from a natural medicine practitioner rather than reading random information on the internet - no matter how credible the information may appear.

I will highlight the supplements that are generally safe and useful for all men. A good multivitamin, and several minerals and vitamins are helpful and safe for almost everyone.

However, some of the supplements that I recommend can be detrimental when taken by a person whose health status is not matched with the way that supplement works.

In this section I give general advice to help you review any supplements you are already taking, and to help prompt a discussion with your practitioner. I strongly recommend that you consult with an experienced natural fertility practitioner before taking any targeted supplements in high dose.

VITAMINS AND MINERALS TO IMPROVE YOUR SPERM

Therapeutic doses of each of the following nutrients are important for achieving good results. However it's not as simple as taking the right dose of a particular nutrient, it's imperative that you get the nutrient in the right form. Sometimes taking a different form will have an inferior effect, sometimes it will have a downright detrimental effect. The clinical outcomes can be wide and varied depending on which form of a particular nutrient you are using. Check labels carefully.

Deficiencies in any one of these can lead to problems with sperm production

Male multivitamin: a general male multivitamin that is practitioner quality will help to fill overall gaps in deficiencies that may be present. Make sure it does not contain either of these two toxic form of b vitamins:

- Folic acid
- Cyanocobalamin

If your multivitamin contains either of these two words on the label - throw it in the bin and replace it with a higher quality product that doesn't contain these toxic ingredients.

Instead of folic acid - look for these ingredients:

- folinic acid
- calcium folinate
- methylfolate
- 5 methyltetrahydrofolate
- quatrefolic
- levomefolate glucosamine
- 5MTHF

Instead of cyanocobalamin - look for these ingredients:

- mecobalamin
- hydroxocobalamin
- methylcobalamin
- adenosylcobalamin

CoQ10: supports mitochondrial energy production and protects against free radical damage. It is shown to improve both athletic performance and recovery, and can also help to improve mitochondrial function. Dosage: 600-900 mg per day. Ubiquinol form is better for more of a "detox" effect. Ubiquinone form is better for supporting mitochondrial function, energy and vitality.

Carnitine: has an antioxidant effect and has been shown to improve motility, count and morphology. Busetto et al. demonstrated the beneficial effect of an antioxidant complex containing carnitine in improving sperm progressive motility compared to baseline. Dosage: 3-6g per day.

Zinc: is a trace mineral essential for normal functioning of the entire male reproductive system. It plays a role in the production of male hormones in the testes. Adequate levels are required to support the process of a sperm being able to penetrate the egg. Zinc acts as a cofactor for more than 200 enzymes in the whole body, including those involved in DNA transcription and protein synthesis. Zinc deficiency is mainly related to low sperm count as measured in the semen parameters, but can also lead to problems with sperm being able to fertilize the egg, and with the longevity of the embryo due to problems with DNA transcription.

Get a blood test to see your baseline levels of zinc. Ask your doctor or natural fertility practitioner for a plasma zinc test. Ideal zinc range is 17-18 mmol/L.

Zinc amino acid chelate and zinc picolinate are the best forms of zinc to increase your zinc status. Dosage: 25mg per day.

Magnesium: helps to improve circulation, vasodilation and nitric oxide production – all these factors help to support sexual arousal and prevent premature ejaculation. It's like mother nature's own Viagra – make sure your magnesium levels aren't low. Magnesium is essential for sperm motility and sperm survival. Ideally this will be in the form of liposomal magnesium, magnesium malate or magnesium amino acid chelate. Magnesium oxide, magnesium sulfate and magnesium chloride are not recommended to support this effect, they primarily have their effect on the digestive system when ingested orally and can lead to diarrhoea. Dosage: 600mg per day up to 800mg per day for people over 80 kg and for those with constipation. Reduce dose if loose bowels occur.

NAC: should be combined with selenium for best effect on improving count, motility and morphology. It supports detoxification by increasing glutathione production, and on its own can be very useful for improving sperm morphology. Dosage: 600mg per day.

Selenium: protects sperm against damage from free radicals, directly and through its role in promoting glutathione production. Is necessary for normal testicular development, sperm production and sperm maturation. Dosage: 250ug per day.

Vitamin E: taken alone or in combination with vitamin C is able to reduce damage to the sperm by free radicals, improve the sperm where DNA fragmentation is present, and improve binding of the spermatozoa to the zona pellucida during the egg fertilization process. Dosage: 500IU per day, ideally with mixed tocotrienols and tocopherols of alpha, beta, gamma and delta.

Vitamin C: often used in combination with vitamin E, is useful for improving all three factors of semen analysis. It can also be useful for improving DNA fragmentation. Dosage: minimum 2g per day, spread across multiple doses.

B Complex: helps with energy levels and also with sperm motility. Activated forms of B vitamins are usually best. Look for supplements that have the following ingredients in the following minimum doses:

- 400ug - 5-MTHF or folinic acid
- 400ug - 1000ug (1mg) - Hydroxocobalamin, Adenosylcobalamin or Methylcobalamin
- 20-40 mg Pyridoxal-5-phosphate (P5P)

Avoid products that contain the following forms of folate and B12:

- Folic acid
- Cyanocobalamin

DO YOU HAVE THE MTHFR MUTATION?

Awareness around MTHFR mutations and their impact on fertility has increased in recent years. However it is only the most progressive practitioners who are testing male partners as well. Knowing the potential MTHFR status of your baby can help you to make more informed decisions about vitamin and mineral supplementation during pregnancy and in the postnatal period. And onwards throughout the duration of your child's life.

It's recommended if you do have MTHFR mutation, especially if you have "compound heterozygous" which is one of each mutation C677T and A1298C, or if you have a double copy of either gene, that you work with a practitioner who understands these genetic mutations and how to optimize your methylation pathways. It's not just a matter of taking a special type of folate or just taking a large dose of folate – it's far more sophisticated than that, and self prescribing or being guided by someone who doesn't fully understand the methylation cycle and how the gene mutations interact can be detrimental to your fertility.

Doctors will often recommend for people with MTHFR C677T mutation to take large doses of folic acid. This recommendation is based on old research. And involves taking a large dose of the toxic form of folate - leading to elevated levels of unmetabolized folic acid in the bloodstream. Unmetabolized folic acid is associated with increased risk of cancer and infertility and should be avoided. Go for the activated form of folate - methylfolate - instead.

ANTIOXIDANTS

A general note about antioxidants is that in many cases, the research around the efficacy of antioxidant supplements is mixed. Antioxidants are best sourced from food and herbal sources rather than from synthetically formulated analogues. Getting a wide range of coloured vegetables will increase your antioxidant intake. There are a number of herbal medicines and super foods that can also help.

Maca: used as a general fertility tonic by South American cultures. Can support testosterone levels.

Goji berries: used traditionally in Chinese medicine to support reproduction, energy levels and vision. Can be useful for men who suffer from lower back pain. Contains beta-carotene and vitamin C among other nutrients.

Resveratrol - is an antioxidant supplement from grapes. It can help to reduce the effects of inflammation on sperm, improves sperm motility, increases testosterone levels and sperm count.

Glutathione – is one of the main detoxifying compounds that the body makes, the liver requires three amino acids and adequate levels of selenium in order to manufacture it. In the absence of these precursors, or if liver function isn't optimal, a glutathione supplement can help to increase levels of glutathione in the body. Some people say that transdermal application of glutathione in a cream, or intravenous glutathione is more effective. Glutathione has positive effects on sperm motility, sperm count and morphology. Men with lower levels of glutathione are more likely to have sperm issues.

Tribulus: has been traditionally used in Ayurvedic medicine as a reproductive tonic to support healthy sexual function and sperm production in men. It should be the Bulgarian variety of tribulus, if the label doesn't state it as Bulgarian, either assume it's not or contact the manufacturer to confirm which species of tribulus they use in their products. Only the Bulgarian variety has potent effects on supporting healthy sexual function. Dosage: 20g per day.

Ashwagandha: is another herb that has been used in Ayurvedic medicine to support healthy sexual function and sperm production in men. It is particularly useful if testosterone levels are low. It has been demonstrated in trials to support increased semen volume, sperm count and motility.

SPECIALTY MALE FERTILITY FORMULAS

These formulas have been used for over a thousand years in the traditions of Chinese herbal medicine and Ayurvedic medicine. When sourcing herbal medicine formulations, it's important to deal with a supplier that uses the highest quality herbs. Pesticide-free and heavy-metal-free organic herbs are especially important to use when you're trying to improve your fertility, and unfortunately herb growers and distributors are just as prone to using synthetic chemicals during their growing and processing as food crops. Organic is best, and go with a trusted brand.

Herbal medicines for fertility are split into two categories: formulas that are specifically for supporting healthy sperm production, and a supportive constitutional formula that helps to enhance the effectiveness of the targeted formula. For best results, these formulas need to be taken together. Using either formula on its own will not be as effective and can impair your results.

(Disclosure: I have a financial interest in Alchemy Herbs, and I use the Alchemy formulas in my clinic with my patients. These are the formulas I have listed below. There are numerous other companies who formulate and dispense Chinese herbal formulas, some you can access without needing a prescription from a practitioner.)

TARGETED FERTILITY FORMULAS

Wild Oats: contains herbs that support the reproductive organs and supports the production of testosterone and spermatogenesis. It's good for men who suffer from fatigue or have aching lower back at the end of the day. This is a useful formula for men who have low sperm count, or low sperm motility.

Smooth: contains herbs that help to improve circulation in the pelvis and is good to use where there are problematic levels of abnormally shaped sperm or if there is low sperm motility. It helps to invigorate blood flow, improve oxygenation, reduce viscosity of the blood, increase vasodilation and nitric oxide production, and has antioxidant properties. Certain types of blockages can be addressed with this formula, which can be useful for low sperm count due to blockage.

Spring Clean: contains herbs that help to improve the clearance of toxins from the body and can also help when there are high levels of abnormally shaped sperm, if there are white cells present in the semen, or if there is agglutination reported in the semen analysis.

Nikki: contains herbs that help to regulate the immune system, and can help when there are elevated levels of sperm antibodies.

Gu formulas: a range of 6 formulas that contain herbs that help to clear out stubborn infections that may be lingering in the pelvis/reproductive area. Contains herbs that simultaneously break down biofilm, clear infection, reduce inflammation, support normal immune response, stimulate cell repair.

MITOCHONDRIAL SUPPORTIVE CONSTITUTIONAL FORMULAS

Warm Me Up: contains herbs that help to improve energy levels and address fatigue, lower back ache, frequent urination, feeling cold, fluid retention (sock marks in lower shins), constipation or loose bowels.

Cool and Moisten: contains herbs that help to improve sleep, improve stress resilience, lower back ache, feeling hot, and constipation.

Relax: contains herbs that help to combat the effects of stress, reduces irritability, reduces headaches, helps with stiff neck, improves digestion, combats fatigue and helps to improve liver function. It's useful for those who are quitting smoking or eliminating their alcohol intake.

SUPPLEMENT QUICK REFERENCE CHART

If you've had a sperm test done, and you know the specific parameters you need to improve upon, the information is summarized here for your easy reference about which supplements might be suitable for you.

	Count	Motility	Morphology
Multivitamin	✓		
Zinc	✓	✓	✓

Selenium	✓	✓	✓
Vitamin A	✓	✓	
Vitamin C	✓	✓	✓
Vitamin E	✓	✓	
B Complex		✓	
Antioxidants	✓	✓	✓
CoQ10	✓	✓	✓
NAC	✓	✓	✓
Magnesium		✓	
Carnitine		✓	
Tribulus	✓	✓	
Wild Oats	✓	✓	
Smooth		✓	✓
Spring Clean			✓
Nikki		✓	✓
Gu Formulas			✓
Warm Me Up	✓	✓	
Cool and Moisten	✓	✓	
Relax		✓	✓

STRATEGIES TO IMPROVE SPERM COUNT

Nutrients like zinc and vitamin C can assist in the production of sperm, but really what is needed is a diet with an abundance of vitamins and minerals. As with the process of making any new cells in the body, adequate rest is needed, so getting good quality sleep, relaxation and doing things that make you happy all contribute to the environment needed in the body to make sperm. If you're taking supplements, zinc should be at least 25–30mg per day, while vitamin C should be taken in four doses of 1g spread across the day.

A magnesium supplement can also help; aim for 200–300 mg twice each day. Powdered magnesium is better absorbed than a tablet; otherwise go for a transdermal magnesium gel or oil. Formulas such as Alchemy Wild Oats (Chinese herbal formula name Wu Zi Yan Zong Wan) and Alchemy Warm Me Up (Chinese herbal formula name You gui Wan) are used as a basis, and are often modified to suit the individual and give best results.

Low sperm count can also be a transport issue, rather than a production issue, so anything that is blocking the passage of sperm out of the testes and into semen can affect the count. It could be the result of an old injury that has damaged the area, or it could be from a varicocele, which is an enlarged vein in the testicle that can block the passage of sperm. Interventions that focus on improving the overall health of the testes can sometimes be useful in helping the body to heal from these problems.

STRATEGIES TO IMPROVE SPERM MORPHOLOGY

Sperm morphology is one of the biggest factors in male subfertility, so this is one part of sperm quality that you don't want to skip over. Zinc is required to make sperm, and a zinc deficiency will often be part of the picture of sperm that have tail defects. Selenium is another nutrient that is required for sperm production and it functions as an anti-oxidant, helping the body to remove any chemicals from the body that could interrupt proper sperm production.

Increasing your intake of leafy green vegetables and increasing your overall nutrition will assist the body to pro-duce better shaped sperm. When the sperm is the right shape, the egg is much more likely to want to accept the sperm. Shape is one of the indicators that allows the egg to know for sure that it's a human sperm.

Reducing exposure to as many chemicals as possible will allow the body space to clear out any excess that is present. Exposure to obvious chemical compounds such as automotive fumes, solvents and paints and chemical waste are not the only sources. In the home, exposure to chemicals comes in the form of shampoo and condition-er, shower gel, shaving cream and aftershave, deodor-ants and antiperspirants, moisturisers, cleaning products, air fresheners and many other products we assume to be "safe".

Many chemical ingredients have the ability to act as endocrine disruptors, interfering with the way your body makes hormones, often acting as estrogen would in the body. In women, these chemicals can lead to a worsen-ing of conditions like PCOS and endometriosis. In men, they can interfere significantly with sperm production and tes-tosterone levels. Cleaning up your home takes a conscious effort over a period of a few months as you replace each product with a less toxic version. Over a fairly short period of time your endocrine system will start to operate more effectively. This is a change that can make a profound difference in a reasonably short period of time, and help to speed up the improvements in sperm morphology.

STRATEGIES TO IMPROVE SPERM MOTILITY

Motility: From a natural medicine point of view the motility is a reflection of the overall state of the man's energy and vitality. This can be seen through any number of observations and symptoms; some of which include a pale tongue, or a tongue with teeth marks on the side, a slow pulse below 60 bpm (yes - even if you're fit, a heart rate below 60 indicates that you have damaged your metabolism), hands, feet or a belly that is cold to touch, general feelings of fatigue, poor digestion (loose bowels or sluggish bowels), and waking from sleep feeling unrefreshed.

Supplements such as Co-enzyme Q10 can be helpful in increasing motility. Others such as B vitamins, zinc and magnesium can also be useful if they are lacking in the diet and a deficiency exists.

Avoiding overexertion is paramount for men with low sperm motility – whether that be overwork, excessive exercise or too much sex – activities that deplete the energy levels will also negatively impact on motility. Use your feelings of wellbeing as a gauge. If you're unsure how to interpret how your energy levels feel from day to day, or you do have low motility but don't feel tired, you can use your basal body temperature as a way to gauge your overall vitality and how it changes from day to day.

Motility is something that can increase and decrease relatively easily, and responds well to changes in diet and lifestyle, improvements to overall nutrition and reduction of stress levels. A range of natural approaches can be useful in helping to improve motility. Making changes to the diet, increasing fluid intake, reducing junk food and processed foods and replacing with fresh fruits and vegetables, small amounts of whole grains and good fats can also help to dramatically improve all sperm factors; as well as mood, energy levels, sleep and general wellbeing. Mayan mas-sage is also something that can be vital to helping to re-align the pelvis and reposition the organs within the pelvis to allow for better blood flow to the prostate and testes.

STRATEGIES TO IMPROVE VARICOCELE

Varicocele is when there are enlarged veins within the scrotum that prevent normal circulation and draining of the testes. They are present in up to 15-20% of men and many have no symptoms. They often evolve over time due to blockage in the veins of the scrotum that leads to a build up of pressure and swelling of the nearby veins. Varicoce-les usually occur on the left side of the scrotum, but can appear on the right side, or less commonly on both sides simultaneously. Symptoms include:

- dragging pain or heaviness of the scrotum

- Vein in the scrotum that is either visible or able to be felt
- Aching pain in the scrotum
- Shrinking of the testicles

The presence of varicocele will reduce testosterone levels, and if varicocele is reversed/treated then testosterone levels will start to return to normal. Increased pregnancy rates in men with treated varicoceles occurs, although not reliably so and some men are better off going for surgical sperm removal from the testes as part of IVF procedure, rather than to attempt varicocele repair.

Varicoceles are more likely to occur in conjunction with a variety of nutritional and lifestyle factors:

- Bowel health
- Smoking status
- Alcohol intake
- Testicular temperature
- Exercise and activity level
- Overstrain due to heavy lifting
- Diet
- Overall health and wellbeing.

There are surgical and non surgical options of varicocele.

Mayan abdominal massage helps to reposition the organs, ligaments and structures of the pelvis to improve blood flow and lymphatic drainage. It can be a useful adjunct to treatment for men with varicocele, and a mayan abdominal massage therapist can teach you the self care massage for you to do at home daily.

Some herbal formulas can be useful for helping to reduce the varicocele. It's important to determine which herbal formula is best suited to use. Using a formula that isn't well suited to the man's constitution can be either not effective, or worsen the problem.

Alchemy Fi (Wen Jing Tang)

- Cold legs or buttocks
- Lower back pain

Alchemy Extinguish (Long dan xie gan tang)

- Liver toxicity due to alcohol intake
- Smoker
- Headaches
- Irritable
- Pimples
- Men who have white blood cells present in semen analysis
- This formula is only for short term use 3-4 weeks maximum

Alchemy Lift Me Up (Bu zhong yi qi tang) – this formula is best suited to men with a history of

- loose bowels
- Fatigue

- Bloating
- poor appetite
- Easy bruising

Men with this grouping of symptoms should work to improve their muscle strength, but do so by using a moderate weight lifting approach only. Heavy lifting in general, and especially a weight training program involving very heavy weights, is detrimental for recovery from this problem.

L-arginine – is used to improve vasodilation and this is vital to helping to undo the underlying cause of the varicocele which in most cases is a blockage within the vein network of the scrotum.

Topically the following herbs will help to improve the strength and integrity of the blood vessels and promote the natural healing of the varicocele:

- Witch hazel
- Butcher's broom
- Horse chestnut
- Yarrow

STRATEGIES TO IMPROVE DNA FRAGMENTATION

Toxicity of chemicals in our modern environment is our biggest enemy against the integrity of DNA, especially in sperm which are the most vulnerable cells in a man's body.

To help reverse DNA fragmentation, we remove the toxins from the body and then allow the new sperm to be formed in an environment that doesn't interfere with DNA integrity. The process takes at least 6 months and involves full detoxification of as many endocrine disrupting chemicals from your body as well as from your household and workplace, in addition to correcting all the factors that impair normal spermatogenesis as described in the main plan.

Focus especially on step 3 of the program – the sperm killers, and on step 6 – the natural medicines that are going to help correct any deficiencies or disharmonies in the body that interfere with normal sperm function.

Castor oil packs on the groin can help to detoxify the chemicals in the local area and improve blood flow, nutrient delivery and oxygenation to the reproductive organs.

STRATEGIES TO IMPROVE SPERM ANTIBODIES

Antibodies are common in men who have had a vasectomy, with up to 75% of these men having sperm antibodies. Men can also form antibodies to their sperm in response to trauma to the testicles: infections such as measles, sports injuries and twisted testicles.

Once the immune system is primed for targeting sperm, a man's body produces antibodies that sit on the head of the sperm and interfere with fertilisation of the egg. There are natural methods to help to reset the immune system so that it no longer treats sperm as foreign cells to be destroyed.

You need to spend six months getting your immune system right. Stopping your immune system from attacking and killing your sperm is only one half of the equation. Once we have your immune system balanced, we then need to start the clock on new sperm production, and we know this takes around 100 days. You should consider this program as a 200 day program to Supercharge Your Sperm to get the full benefits. Some men need to spend up to 12 months or even longer in order to reduce their sperm antibodies to a level that allows pregnancy to occur.

There are five key factors to addressing sperm antibodies:

- getting the immune system cofactors in place: selenium, zinc, vitamin C
- harmonizing the immune system: getting gut dysbiosis sorted out, identifying allergies and other immune irritants in your diet, home or workplace
- ensuring all aspects of your body are functioning in harmony to help reduce inflammation in the body
- reducing stress, which is one of the key factors in regulating the immune system
- opening up blood and lymph flow throughout the pelvic area to optimize healing time.

STRATEGIES FOR OVER 40s

The chance of conceiving with IVF once either partner is above the age of 40 declines pretty quickly. The risk of infertility, and miscarriage increases with the age of the male partner, or the female partner. In addition, the drugs used to stimulate the ovaries for the egg collection process require the woman to be a long way away from menopause because they are the same hormones (FSH, Follicle Stimulating Hormone) that start to increase as a woman nears menopause.

Although it can become more challenging to successfully harvest eggs once you are in your 40s (or as your FSH starts to increase), the decline in the chances of conceiving naturally does not happen until several years after your FSH begins to creep up. The main focus at this age is to ensure that your partner is ovulating each month. Provided ovulation is happening and she does not have blocked tubes, your chance of conceiving naturally is comparable to IVF and in many cases is higher.

However, this relies on your sperm being in top shape – they have to fertilize her egg the old fashioned way. This means they have to swim the whole way, they need the endurance and longevity to make the journey, and have the vitality once there to be able to penetrate her egg to fertilize it.

Achieving pregnancy into your 40s is all about reaching optimum health. Peak fertility and good genetic expression occur when the body is in a state of balance, and it is here that your biological age matters more than your chronological age. Chronological age is the number of years you've been on the planet – that's the part that we can't change. But just because you're "over the hill" and over the age of 40, it doesn't mean you have to resign yourself to the scrap heap. There are plenty of "young" 42-year-olds, likewise there are many "old" 32-year-olds, and the fertility of someone who is taking care of themselves in a way that manifests as a youthful appearance, energy, vitality and vigour will be stronger than it would be otherwise. The saying "Live fast, die young" applies just as much to your reproductive potential – if you live a stressful and not life-sustaining or life-respecting existence, then your reproductive potential will die off much earlier than it would do otherwise. Dialling things back, reducing stress, really taking care of yourself and creating an optimal environment within your body is important for anyone considering conceiving, but it is the most crucial aspect of the program for those over 40.

I cannot stress this enough. As much as you are capable, take on board lifestyle and diet changes that support you to be as youthful, energetic, refreshed and vital as possible. This program is perfect for helping you to regain your energy and restore your vitality. If you follow it, you are giving yourselves the best chances of conceiving.

Also on the non-negotiable list is that both of you need to be fully engaged in a comprehensive program that involves 12 months of solid commitment and dedication to your health and lifestyle. Because you are older, there is more work to be done to wind back the negative effects the modern lifestyle has had on your fertility.

Think of this program more as a 12 month plan, and even consider which aspects you will retain in the long term, even beyond the time that you are considering fertility and baby-making. Some couples may conceive sooner than 12 months, some take longer than this. I always remind my patients, these strategies aren't just for improving your fertility, they are strategies for improving your overall health and wellbeing, your quality of life, and the connection, intimacy and resilience in your relationship.

ACTION PLAN

1. Check the labels on any supplements you are currently taking. Do they contain folic acid or cyanocobalamin? If so - throw them away and replace them with better quality supplements.

2. Review any supplements you are taking to see if you are taking a therapeutic dose, and to ensure you are taking the best bioavailable form of each nutrient. You may need to adjust your dosage or get a new product to replace an inferior product you have already been taking.

3. Check your sperm test results to see which parameters you need to focus on (refer to chapter 6 for how to read your results). Choose supplements that are going to help target the areas you need to work on.

4. Consider working in conjunction with a natural fertility practitioner, they are the experts in knowing which supplements are going to be most beneficial for you. An experienced practitioner can prescribe a program for you that will take into account all the factors that need to be addressed to optimize your health and improve your sperm production.

STEP 7: STAYING ON TRACK

You are now well and truly into the program. Which changes have you already implemented? How are you feeling? If you have already implemented most of the changes over a period of a few weeks or more - are you noticing the benefits? Do you have more energy? Have you noticed a change in your body shape? Your complexion? Are you getting unsolicited comments from friends or work colleagues that you are looking younger/fitter/healthier?

Whilst the reason you are undertaking this program is not to get compliments from the people you interact with on a regular basis, it is nice to get feedback that the hard work you have put in is paying off.

So well done on getting this far.

But - it takes 100 days for sperm to be made from start to finish, and now is a great time to double down on your why. Why are you doing this program? Why is it important to you to be improving your health, improving your fertility? Perhaps go back and re-read chapter 1 if you are starting to feel complacent, and contemplating letting old habits creep back in.

Don't be tempted by a morning coffee if you're feeling flat. Drink 2 large glasses of water first thing in the morning instead, to hydrate you. Follow this with a decent breakfast and get your metabolism going. You'll have energy in no time.

Stay strong with your efforts in avoiding alcohol. By now you've probably already survived at least one social outing where you didn't drink. Keep it up for the other events that you'll come up against in the next couple of months.

You might be doing totally fine. And have really good momentum with your new habits. It only takes around a month to reprogram yourself into new habits and new ways of thinking, so you've already done all the hard work. Maintaining your new changes is the only challenge here.

The way to make it easy for yourself, and to help these changes stay firmly in place for the rest of this 100 day program and beyond, is to focus on the prize. Imagine how you might feel when you see those two lines showing up on a pregnancy test to say that your partner is pregnant. Imagine how you might feel when you see your baby for the first time on ultrasound. Imagine how it might feel to hold your baby in your arms for the first time.

These are the thoughts and feelings that will make it easy for you to stay on track. Remind yourself that you aren't just making these changes for yourself. You will definitely benefit. Your relationship with your partner will benefit. Your child will reap the rewards with the best possible foundations for good health and vitality throughout their life.

TIME TO RE-EVALUATE

You have had time now to implement all the logistical changes that are involved in the program. By now you're starting to settle into your routines with eating, exercising, and relaxation. So it's the perfect time for us to re-evaluate your current health status, to see if any changes have occurred.

Primarily we need to assess how you are going as a couple – how is your relationship after embarking on the program? Now that you are doing more things together – eating well, exercising, focusing on intimacy and communication, have you noticed that you are getting along better with each other? Do you feel closer to her?

The SuperSperm Checklist - have any of these symptoms improved for you in the past month?

- Fatigue
- Feel flat or low mood (including depression)
- Use reflux or antacid medication
- Use asthma medication
- Losing hair, or starting to go grey
- Aching or pain in the lower back
- Sweat at night in bed
- Digestion isn't great
- Loss of morning erections

Optimal Health Checklist - have any of these additional symptoms improved for you in the past month?

- Sleep
- Skin
- Headaches
- Appetite
- Your ability to achieve and maintain an erection

A lot of men notice improvements in multiple areas of their health, even in areas of their health that they didn't think they had a problem with.

However there may still be areas of your health that *haven't* improved since embarking on this program - this could indicate that you need additional support either from your natural fertility practitioner, or your doctor.

KICKING GOALS AND REACHING TARGETS

Any plan that is worth following should have a way for you to measure that you're on track. And if you've fallen off track, have a way for you to get back on target. Know the markers that you're looking for when it comes to tracking your overall health and your fertility.

By the time you're 2 months in to the program, many men are experiencing noticeable improvements to their overall health and vitality.

Once you've been following the program for 2 months, revisit the checklists to see how you are doing:

The SuperSperm Checklist - have any of these symptoms improved for you in the past 2 months?

- Fatigue
- Feel flat or low mood (including depression)
- Use reflux or antacid medication
- Use asthma medication
- Losing hair, or starting to go grey
- Aching or pain in the lower back
- Sweat at night in bed
- Digestion isn't great
- Loss of morning erections

Optimal Health Checklist - have any of these additional symptoms improved for you in the past 2 months?

- Sleep
- Skin
- Headaches
- Appetite
- Your ability to achieve and maintain an erection

DO YOU NEED EXTRA MOTIVATION?

If you are finding that you need extra help and motivation, the benefits of working with a natural health practitioner can be invaluable in helping to keep you on track.

Now that you're two thirds of the way through the program, you are well aware by now of the parts of the program that you find easy and enjoyable. And also if there are any parts of the program that you wish were easier for you to enjoy.

The first step in staying motivated is acknowledging how well you are sticking to the program. Identify the parts of the program that you enjoy, and find easy - and really focus for a moment on how that feels for you. Feel the sense of achievement, and joy and pride and whatever other positive emotions you associate with your success in those areas of the program.

Now let's try to create those same feelings around the parts of the program that feel challenging for you. Can you identify exactly what it is that's stopping you from feeling the same way about all the aspects of the program? What do you need in order to be able to feel like you can enjoy all parts of the program?

One way to stay motivated is to set smaller goals for yourself each week. Perhaps you and your partner could engage in some friendly competition if that suits your relationship dynamic. Setting down a challenge to help breathe some life into the parts of the program you find more challenging can help you to stay on track.

Another way is to get an accountability buddy. Enlist a friend who you can go to the gym with. Or find a friend who will go with you to meditation classes. Start an instagram challenge with your friends to post your healthy meals every day for a week, or a month. It's often easier for us to stick to our plans if we feel accountable to another person other than ourselves.

ACTION PLAN

1. Reflect on changes in your relationship. Are you happy with the way things are going now between you? Are there ways you could develop further closeness and intimacy without the pressure of sex attached?

2. If there are aspects of your health that still aren't quite where you'd like them to be, visit your natural fertility practitioner or your GP to discuss any further testing or treatment that might be necessary.

3. Re-read the chapter and follow the steps to identify the parts of the program that you enjoy and find easy, and the parts of the program you find challenging.

4. Try to identify several strategies that could help you to enjoy all the aspects of the program. It might be booking a regular class, it could be finding an accountability buddy. Find ways to make the program fun.

5. Keep revisiting this exercise if you need to overcome any bad habits that have started to creep back in.

6. If you haven't already signed up for the program emails with the hints, tips and reminders - do this at clarepyers.com/supercharge so that you can be supported in staying motivated for the remainder of the program.

PART III:
WHAT HAPPENS NEXT?

O nce you have made it through your first 3 months of the program - congratulations! You have been on the program long enough to have made a measurable improvement to multiple markers of your health and fertility! Well done!

Before you go and plan a massive feast filled with all the foods and alcohol that you have been avoiding since starting this program, take a moment to reflect on how you feel.

How are your energy levels now? Do you feel younger and more vibrant?

How is your mood?

Has your weight or body shape changed?

Has your libido improved?

How is your relationship with your partner?

Whether you and your partner are pregnant now or not, think about all the benefits that you have gained from these new habits of looking after yourself in every way. How many of these benefits would you like to continue to experience in your life, going forward? Would you like to have high levels of energy continue through your partner's pregnancy and through to the early stages of parenthood where fatigue and sleep deprivation will be thrust upon you?

Which parts of the program will you continue to have as your new default approach to life?

Don't give up the fruits of your efforts just yet. It's easier to sustain these improvements, than it is to let them slide and then try to start again at a later date. Keep as many parts of the program in your regular routine as you can, and it will serve to keep you healthy and with enough energy to live the life you want to live.

BONUS CHAPTER 1:
PREGNANT!

Congratulations! You're pregnant. But you're not over the line yet.

Unfortunately one in four pregnancies will end in miscarriage and so we need to make sure that your body is prepared and remains in good condition in the unfortunate circumstance that you might lose the baby and are back trying for another baby in a few months time.

The other reason that you don't want to take your foot off the pedal just yet is that it's going to work really well for you if you can stay in peak physical condition. Your role in this equation of making a new family or expanding your existing family is more than just simply being a sperm donor, you're one half of the adult population of your household and very much required in terms of the running of the household. Most importantly, you're the main support person for your partner. Dropping the ball now and returning to some of your old habits – maybe eating some take-away food or having a few drinks with the boys or losing your momentum with exercise – is going to decrease your overall state of health and well-being and mean that you're not going to be able to have the energy levels or the motivation to be able to support your partner when you know she probably needs it the most.

THE FIRST TRIMESTER

When a woman is in her first trimester of pregnancy, quite often she's tired and also feeling unwell. She probably doesn't want to do a lot of cooking and her nose will be quite sensitive to smells, so cleaning products will be diffi-cult for her to use right now. The majority of the housework and tasks around the house are going to fall into your lap as her body is trying to make the contribution towards es-tablishing the pregnancy.

There can also be a lot of anxiety around the early stag-es of pregnancy with women feeling cautious and some-times quite nervous that there is the possibility of losing the pregnancy. You can be a really valuable support person for her at this time and help her to connect with what's actu-ally going on in her body so that she's not so focused on the things that might be going wrong but more focused on what she's feeling that's different. You've probably al-ready noticed an increase in the size of her breasts, there can also be a change in vaginal discharge; there are so many changes that are happening in her body. From a metabolism point of view, a pregnant woman is running the equivalent of a marathon everyday, this is the amount of effort that is needed in the early stages of pregnancy in order to be able to establish, maintain and support a growing fetus. So there's a lot of energy that's going into that and there's not a lot left over at the end of the day for providing interesting conversation, let alone cooking and cleaning and doing other tasks around the house – make sure to really show how much you are able to take care of.

One of the things that makes a really big difference in the first trimester is the amount of rest that a pregnant woman gets. Studies have been done on women with multiple prior miscarriages – a rate as high as 80% – and what they found is that when these women are taught how to meditate and relax and are given time off work, so they are resting more and not doing as much activity, the rate of miscarriage can reduce to 15-20% which is the average miscarriage rate in the population. So don't discount her need to rest, relax and avoid stress. As far as arguments go – save it for another time if you can so that her stress hormone levels can remain as balanced as possible.

THE SECOND TRIMESTER

The start of the second trimester marks a time where miscarriage risk is greatly reduced, and many couples are now revealing their exciting news to their wider circle of family, friends and colleagues.

Women who experience nausea and vomiting in the first trimester often feel relief once they are in the second trimester. Their energy can start to pick up and generally this is a time when women feel their best during pregnancy.

This is a time for you to enjoy each other again and reconnect if you started to feel a little disconnected in the early stages of her pregnancy. It's still relatively easy for her to forget about being pregnant, which makes it a great time to think about taking trips away, or doing other social activities like going to a concert or a show.

Around the 20 week mark, she will already be feeling the baby move, and if you stay close to her with your hand on her tummy you will be able to feel the baby move and kick. It's a special feeling to experience, and a good way for you to spend quality time together, connecting with each other, dreaming about how life will be when you get to meet your baby.

THE THIRD TRIMESTER

As a woman makes it to the third trimester her belly is really showing, and the physical reality of having a second per-son growing in her body is starting to show. Moving around can start to be more uncomfortable for her, finding a com-fortable sleeping position can be difficult, she may start to develop back or hip pain. Everything will start to take her longer to do, if your partner is a woman who likes to whiz around and get lots of things done in a short period of time, you may notice that she takes considerably longer to do things than she did in the past.

Now is a great time to step things up and take over the lion's share of household tasks and other things that require heavy lifting and effort. Doing grocery shopping, cleaning, moving furniture to set up the baby's new room.

The baby is getting quite large now - pushing on her internal organs and making it difficult for her to eat in the same way as before. If you have a routine of eating togeth-er - try doing things in sync with her and have half your dinner earlier in the evening than normal, and the second half of your dinner together at the regular time. One of the most common and preventable issues of the third trimes-ter is reflux, eating smaller meals more regularly is an easy way to reduce this symptom for a lot of pregnant women. Avoid trigger foods - starchy carbs like pasta and potato, chilli, curries and coffee are all common culprits when it comes to reflux. Explore with her different food options that can help her to overcome this problem if it arises.

PREPARING FOR BIRTH

By this stage, most women are tired, weary and mentally worn out from being pregnant. Many women are keen to meet their baby, and keen to get their body back - and to experience their body without a person on the inside rest-ing on their internal organs.

A lot of physical discomfort can arise because of the way her body has changed so dramatically - tightness in her upper back and between the shoulder blades is very common. As is tightness and discomfort in the lower back and hips. Help with any lower back ache she might be ex-periencing, and also help to loosen the muscles and liga-ments around her hips and pelvis. Having supple muscles around the hips and pelvis helps make for easier birthing for her, there is less resistance coming from her body as her pelvis expands to let the baby through during labour. Mas-sage is really easy to learn, there are some great videos on my website showing you how to massage your partner to connect you together.

Massaging her back, hips and pelvis can provide enormous relief to her - and it's good practice for your hands to get used to massaging her in the leadup to birth. Massaging her lower back and sacrum during delivery can provide very effective pain relief during the early stages of labour - the more practice and stamina in your hands you can build during these weeks, the better equipped you will be to support her during birth.

POST-NATAL PERIOD (THE FOURTH TRIMESTER)

Your baby is here, and you are in awe of your partner for the amazing job she has done in providing her body as a vessel to grow and nurture this amazing little human. How great that you get to meet your new baby! And you are just so in love with both these special people in your life.

Then the reality sets in - this new little person needs milk, lots of it, and very frequently. And your partner is exhausted, and trying to navigate the massive changes in her body. Neither of you feel like you're getting sleep. Her abdomen, the space where just a few days ago she had a little person growing in there, now feels empty and hollow over the next few weeks as everything tries to rearrange itself back how it was before. She may have mixed feelings about her body, and the way that it is or isn't going back to the shape she hoped for. Be sensitive to this, everyone will be showering attention on the baby, you can take this opportunity to also shower attention on her and the fantastic job she has done.

The good news is that with all the preparation you put into your health in the leadup to pregnancy, you are now in good stead to be dealing with this taxing time. It's easier to get through your days if your energy levels are already high. It's easier to deal with sleep deprivation and the stress it causes on your body, if you have continued with your good eating habits, exercise and meditation routine. Keep it up now, cooking meals to provide valuable nourishment to all three of you, so she can rest in between feeding the baby. Keep a good stock of healthy snacks and ready made meals in the house so she can replenish herself as needed (breastfeeding is hard work and requires lots of calories). Soon you'll get into a routine, and before you know it the weeks will pass, the months will pass and then you'll be back to the start - contemplating whether or not you'll have another baby. Then you can start this 7 step program again!

BONUS CHAPTER 2:
WHEN TO STOP TRYING

There is no right or wrong answer on when it's the right time to stop trying for a baby. There are many options available to couples who are willing to invest time, money and effort into comprehensive testing, cutting edge IVF treatments, and those who want to cover all the bases of removing as many barriers as possible to conceiving.

SUCCESS RATES

Despite all these advances in technology, and all the wonderful things we can do with mainstream medicine, cutting edge science, natural medicine, and the fusion of these modalities, there is no approach that has a 100% success rate. Nobody can guarantee you a baby.

IVF clinics will often cite their statistics on age groups, these can be as high as 30-40% in younger couples, and as low as 5% for couples over the age of 40. What most IVF clinics don't reveal is that the chance of you getting pregnant can vary greatly depending on which specialist you are seeing, and within the same centre your chances of getting pregnant could be more than double if you are with one specialist rather than another. Clinical experience, a willingness to try new treatments, as well as intuition can play a role. So if you've been unsuccessful with one fertility specialist, another fertility specialist in the same clinic, or in a different clinic, may be able to provide fresh insights into your treatment that could make a difference.

THE TOLL OF IVF

In Australia there is currently no limit to the number of government subsidised IVF cycles a couple can undertake. I've spoken with many couples who are reluctant to stop trying, feeling like a successful pregnancy could be just one IVF cycle away. Even with financial subsidy, the out of pocket expenses can be substantial, and it is not unheard of for couples to spend upwards of $100,000 on IVF and still not have a baby to take home with them. In other countries, there isn't the same access to subsidised IVF treatment, and so couples are either limited in the number of cycles they can do, or they are limited by their financial capacity to pay the full cost of treatment. In Australia, especially when pursuing treatment at a fully funded medicare bulk billing clinic, it's a couple's emotional resilience, and a woman's physical ability to withstand the effects of treatment that are the limiting factors on the number of cycles a couple will undertake. Often I am working with couples who have already had a number of failed cycles, and I am seeing them when they are already at the point of emotional exhaustion.

STRONGER RELATIONSHIP

This program could be your starting point on your fertility journey and much of this terminology could be foreign to you.

Or - you may already be very familiar with many of the terms and concepts in this book. You and I may be meeting each other for the first time as you're reading this book, once you are already well and truly a long way into your fertility journey. This program may be your last hope.

No matter which point you are at, one of the benefits of you and your partner embarking on this program together, and experiencing these changes together is that your relationship will be stronger. The two of you are a team, much more so than you were before. You've taken on a project of getting healthy together, working towards a common goal, reconnecting with each other, dealing with your stress more effectively. These are the ingredients for a strong relationship that can withstand the upset and disappointment of not getting pregnant.

LIFE WITHOUT KIDS

Will you adopt? Would you consider surrogacy? Will you be a fabulous uncle and aunt to your nieces and nephews, or the kids from next door? There can be other ways to fulfil the parenting instincts in your life, that don't involve your partner being pregnant.

Maybe you will implement plan B and redesign the way your next 20 - 30 years of life might play out.

Fertility counselors are highly skilled at supporting and guiding you through the decisions you would like to make around your fertility. They can help you find the answer that is right for you around when to stop trying, and how to navigate your feelings around surrogacy, adoption, or a life without your own children if this is what you will choose.

CONCLUSION

Fertility problems can take a toll on a couple's relationship. The woman usually shoulders the entirety of the blame, and the burden of seeking assistance in overcoming the barriers to you getting pregnant.

She feels more and more isolated, and alone, and your relationship can suffer as the distance between you grows. She's putting in so much effort, going to appointments, reading up online on the latest fertility supplement, and the things she can do to improve the chances of conceiving.

Meanwhile, without any information or dialog about things you can be doing to help the process along, you, her partner, her hero, her king, are sitting by and watching helplessly as the months go past and a positive pregnancy test remains elusive. The woman you love, the woman you want to have babies with, is devastated, beyond upset, and so disappointed that her body has let her down, and continues to let her down month after month. And she continues on this journey of self improvement alone, making sacrifices whilst you're out drinking with friends. And your relationship starts to suffer as the distance between you, and the frustration and resentment builds.

What if there was something you could do that could make a difference? Something that you can do to show her that you are on her side. Something you can do that could also help to improve your fertility, and improve the quality and vitality of your sperm and make it more likely you will conceive. Something that you could do that would improve your quality of life in every aspect - your health, your relationship.

That was the reason for me writing this book. To get couples on the same page, to remind them of their shared goals, and remind them how to work together as a team towards their dream of becoming parents. Too often I encounter women in my clinic who are in tears, sobbing at the lack of support from their partner when it comes to their fertility journey.

Too often I discussed with men what they would be willing to do in order to help alleviate their partner's suffering. Most men would be willing to do anything. They just didn't know what they could do that would make a difference. Most men love the idea of being her knight in shining armor, and being the hero of the story.

This 7 step program is the result of me trying to summarize the clinical approach I take with my male patients. Summarize the coaching steps I work through with my patients and offer strategies to help you overcome the common hurdles and obstacles I see patients encounter.

Working with men over the years, I have seen the way that their female partners glow and beam and are brought back to life when their partners are working with me. They see the positive changes that occur, they feel supported, they feel like a team again. This was one of the biggest surprises to me, and one of the best side effects of a program that originally was just designed to help improve a man's fertility and boost a couple's chances of getting pregnant.

The program involves making a number of big diet and lifestyle changes, not for the faint of heart, but we're talking big stakes here. This program could be the difference between you being able to conceive or not. Of course, it's not a guarantee that you'll end up with a baby, however, improving your overall health prior to conceiving is part of the equation of having the healthiest child you possibly can. And in the meantime you are strengthening your relationship, falling back in love with one another, and improving your health and vitality in the process too.

I sincerely hope you have enjoyed reading this book, and find it to be useful in supporting you and your partner in your fertility journey.

Best wishes to you both.

Clare Pyers

RESOURCES

This book is not an academic piece. It is a book primarily written for my patients, based on my 20 years (so far) of clinical experience. The references and resources that were available at the time I first started writing this book over 7 years ago have changed so drastically that some of them are almost now obsolete. There are so many studies that have been published in that 7 year period that have added so much richness to the information we now have about infertility that it's just not possible to do justice by adding here a list of journal articles and research papers for you to look at.

On my website, I have collated an up-to-date list of research papers investigating various aspects of both male and female infertility. You can find this information at:

https://clarepyers.com/fertility-research

WORK WITH ME

I sincerely hope you feel inspired to make changes to your life now that you have read this book. The purpose of writing this book was to be able to reach far more people than I have the ability to see in my private consulting practice.

If you feel called to reach out to me and work with me one-on-one in implementing the information in this book, please do so. I work with patients all over the world, via tele-health and in-person consults at my clinic is Melbourne, Australia. You can find out more about booking consults with me on my website:

https://clarepyers.com

I look forward to working with you!

www.ingramcontent.com/pod-product-compliance
Lightning Source LLC
Chambersburg PA
CBHW062054270326
41931CB00013B/3067